A Guide to Classic Discipline

By Morgan Thorne

A Guide to Classic Discipline
Copyright © 2017 Morgan Thorne
Second Edition, 2017
ISBN 978-0-9958780-0-6
www.MsMorganThorne.com

Published by:
Nymphetamean Publishing
www.Nymphetamean.com
Toronto, Ontario

Booksellers: For best results, display in the Sexuality section.

Warning & Disclaimer: This book is intended to be a reference guide and leaning aid. It is not a complete education on BDSM. The author strongly advises that people get in person instruction from an experienced instructor prior to engaging in BDSM activities.
The author and publisher assume no responsibilities for any injuries, loss, or damages resulting from the ideas presented in this book. The practice of BDSM comes with significant risks and while these can be lessened, they still exist. The use of drugs or alcohol greatly increases these risks. By acting on the information in this book, you assume all responsibility for your actions

For Sage, my wonderful partner. This book wouldn't be
possible without your love and support.
Thank you for keeping me motivated.
Even when I didn't want to be.

Contents

Introduction

Classic Discipline has many names in BDSM; Old Fashioned Discipline, The English Arts, Judicial Discipline, to name a few. It covers a wide range of activities, from sensual to severe, and is often what we think of when we think about punishments and play.

Frequently, our first introduction to kink is a simple slap on the ass. This innocent gesture can lead down the wonderful path of BDSM to much more sensual and severe kinky play. Many of us get our start with this informal introduction to kink by a lover. A little horse-play with our lovemaking opens the door to something inside our minds that we didn't know was there. Perhaps we read some racy fan fiction or other hot and steamy story that incorporated some slap and tickle with the bump and grind, our minds lingering on the hotness of the kink instead of the rest of the story.

Some of us have always known we were different. When discovering our sexuality, we may have stumbled on something we saw as darker, an urge to hurt or be hurt. In the age of the internet, it's easier to find resources on BDSM. Before that, we may have found ourselves lucky with a more experienced kinky lover. We may have also hidden our desires for fear of our partner's reaction.

However you ended up here, this book intends to be an introduction to the themes of Classic Discipline for both play and punishment. You will learn about the history of the style, the implements, get ideas on how to incorporate elements into your play style or how to run whole scenes in this style. We will draw inspiration from around the world and from history as we evoke some stark imagery of punishment that will strike fear into the hearts of bottoms and inspire Tops with a sense of power.

Classic Discipline has its roots in the British school and judiciary systems, so much of the imagery and implements are drawn from this point in history. Classic Discipline can also draw influence from the unsavoury traditions of corporal punishment of various countries throughout the world. The 1950's tend to be a big influence on the world of Classic Discipline, with many of the practitioners growing up seeing this depiction of 'the good life' on television and in pop culture. Finally, Classic Discipline can also incorporate elements of childhood punishments; things which evoke those deep rooted memories of our younger years.

Some people will be drawn to a specific style of discipline, others will pick and choose elements from many traditions, bringing them together to create their own unique style. Some styles of discipline are better suited for a particular scene or can evoke a mood or feeling, so feel free to use what suits your goals.

Terms Used in This Book

When it comes to BDSM, the terms we use have fairly loose definitions - everyone has their own version. For the sake of clarity, I want to explain which terms I've chosen to use, why and what they mean in the context of this book. This way, we can all be on the same page and hopefully avoid potential confusion or offence.

In the course of this book, I've tried to use gender-neutral terms as much as possible. I've used "they" or "them" as pronouns as opposed to gendered terms because dominance (and by extension submission) doesn't belong to any specific gender. Gender itself is such a fluctuating, evolving and non-binary concept.

I've also decided to use the words "Top" and "bottom" throughout most of the book because many of the activities I will be describing do not require any sort of power exchange. I will be using "Top" to describe the person who is doing the action - the person administering the spanking, for example. "Bottom" describes the person on the receiving end of the action - the person being spanked.

In parts of the book where I am describing power exchange specifically, I will use "Dominant" and "submissive". For clarity, the Dominant is the one directing the action, who has the authority, the submissive is the one following direction, who cedes to the Dominant's authority. I have avoided terms like "Dom" or "Domme" because they carry assumptions of gender that aren't useful for us in this context.

While I haven't written specifically about switching in the context of discipline, I encourage switches to take what they want from the book and apply it as they see fit. In fact, I encourage everyone of whichever orientation or label to take what they find useful and discard the rest.

I have used a number of acronyms, for the sake of brevity. I have tried to stick with acronyms that are fairly common in the kink world so that there is as little confusion as possible. The first instance has the full words, and subsequent references will use the acronym only.

For instance, power exchange, the activity of giving up or taking power in a consensually negotiated way, is shortened to "PE". Total power exchange, a way to describe a relationship style where the submissive gives up all authority to the Dominant, is shortened to "TPE". The relationship between a Dominant and submissive is shortened to "D/s". Other abbreviations used in the book will be indicated on their first use.

Now that we are hopefully on the same page, let's take a look at the history of Classic Discipline and how we got to this point with BDSM.

History of Classic Discipline

Erotic pain has a long and rich history, that stretches back as far as people have been recording such things. We can find evidence of it throughout history, showing that not only did ancient people have a penchant for discipline but they also had a liking for pornography!

From the Tomb of the Whipping in the Necropolis of Monterozzi near Tarquinia, Italy we see frescos from approximately 490 BC. Most notably one of two men whipping a woman bent over between them. The painting is badly damaged, but it doesn't take much imagination to guess what she might be doing with her head near the one man's groin, the other man with his hand on her ass, whip raised all of them stark naked.

The Kama Sutra is probably the most famous book on human sexuality ever written, despite its ancient origins. It is believed to be composed between 400 BCE and 200 CE, written in Sanskrit, it covers all aspects of love, family life and other things which are needed in the pursuit of a virtuous life - which includes physical pleasure and intimacy shared with a loved one. The chapters which provide advice on sexual congress also offer advice on how to apply pain as a part of lovemaking - through biting, marking with nails, striking with the hands and more. These acts are described as consensual, erotic and to enhance the pleasure felt by the people involved, not with the intention to inflict harsh pain.

If the Kama Sutra is the most famous book on human sexuality, the Marquis de Sade is the most famous historical pervert and pornographer. Born June 2, 1740, and died December 2, 1814, Donatien Alphonse François de Sade, the Marquis, spent nearly 32 years of his life in various prisons and asylums because of his inflammatory and perverse writings; both erotic and political. De Sade was well known for his love of prostitutes, however, many of them complained of abuse - complaints that were echoed by many of his servants and others in de Sade's employ. He was charged many times in his life, spending time in prison, asylums and escaping from both, using his nobility and money to shirk responsibility and shift blame to others. It always bothers me when kinksters call him the 'grandfather of s/m' since he often acted without consent and without regard to the boundaries or feelings of his victims.

Around the same time, other books combining pain and pleasure were written. John Cleland's Fanny Hill was published in 1749. Brothels specializing in flagellation and other erotic pain practices were well known by the mid to late 1700's, perhaps capitalizing on the self-flagellation rituals of the church during the medieval era.

The BDSM we know and love is a more modern movement, that likes to romanticize the past. In the early part of the 20th century was the first of three defining principles of modern kink as described by Robert Bienvenu. European Fetish was at its height in pre world war two Germany, well known for being sexually progressive. American Fetish took shape during the depression in the US and was in full swing by 1934. It helped shape many of the iconic fetish items we have today, including high heels, long gloves, uniforms and human ponies. Modern BDSM was further shaped by the rise of the Gay Leather scene. Taking fashion cues from biker culture, the Gay Leather scene provided a structured and alternative expression of gay male sexuality.

The 1960's saw a loosening of sexual mores, for vanilla and kinky alike. Bettie Page became a BDSM idol and still inspires many today. She became the first famous bondage model through her work with Irving Klaw. Shooting both 8mm film and still photographs, Klaw produced highly fetishistic images of Page as both Dominatrix and submissive for his clientele.

Eric Stanton also worked with Klaw, drawing bondage cartoons for Klaw's publication 'Movie Star News'. He also self-published books of his work known as Stantoons. His most memorable characters were Blunder Broad, a super-heroine who found herself often captured, tortured and stripped of her superpowers by cunnilingus; and various Prinkazons, giant women who grew huge penises and loved to humiliate men with face sitting, scat play, and anal rape.

John Willie produced Bizarre Magazine from 1946 to 1959, showcasing a wide variety of kinky activities but often focused on cross-dressing and gender-bending. He also made famous the 'G-String Tie' which is said to be very difficult to escape from.

The 1970s and 1980s saw a growing underground BDSM culture. In the 1970s when some feminists were disparaging kink, a group of kinky nomadic lesbians (no, I'm not making that up) known as the Van Dykes were discovering and enjoying power play and sadomasochism. The 70s also saw a surge in Nazi themes. Films such as 'The Night Porter' and 'Ilsa, She Wolf of the SS' were cult hits. Penthouse Magazine featured an SM themed photo set with a man dressed as an SS officer.

A documentary on BDSM called 'S/M: One Foot Out of the Closet' was aired by KQED (Public Media for Northern California) in 1980. The film interviewed a number of people of different sexual orientations - their identities obscured - and found them to be fairly normal. Straight couples would frequent gay bars as one of the few places they could go to be publicly kinky.

The 80s also saw the start of the Folsom Street Fair in San Francisco. It is the longest running and largest BDSM gathering of it's kind, going into its 33rd year (as of the writing of this book). It has inspired other similar events, including Folsom East in New York City, Folsom Europe in Berlin and Folsom North in Toronto.

The internet opened BDSM communities and culture up for mass consumption. It makes kinky gatherings and information much easier to find for the curious and fed into popular culture's need to be outraged and titillated (preferably at the same time).

Web sites such as Fetlife, Alt.com, and CollarSpace made finding other kinky people easier. Pop stars began to incorporate fetish attire into their wardrobes. Television commercials play with BDSM stereotypes for laughs. Of course, the 50 Shades of Grey books brought swarms of excited people out to kink events. Many found that some fantasies are better off as fantasies, while others...Well, maybe you're reading this now.

Historical Discipline, Modern Kink

With that relatively brief understanding of the history of BDSM, let's move on to a brief history of the discipline styles that we will be discussing in this book. For some, my history lesson may be enough to get a feel for the discipline tradition in question. For others, this will be a jumping off point for further research with the goal of the most realistic and genuine interpretation of historical discipline they can manage.

Naval Discipline

When we talk about Naval Discipline, we are generally referring to the British Navy. At one point it was the largest naval fleet in the world and was notorious for its strict, uncompromising discipline. Many of the sailors were not there willingly, so quick and severe punishment was needed to keep things running smoothly. The height of this harsh regime was the 17th century through to the early 19th century. Flogging with cat-o-nine tails was a common and brutal punishment that was finally banned in the 1880's. Caning and other forms of corporal punishment were used until 1949 when it was formally banned.

The Articles of War detailed the various crimes and penalties for sailors. They were drilled into every man, read aloud each week by the captain to all crew members. Punishments varied depending on the age of the accused - children were chastised in slightly less extreme ways than adults. Boys were often flogged on the bare bottom, whereas men received their lashes on the bare back. Of course, adults would sometimes be punished as children if it was deemed they were 'too big for their boots'.

Serious crimes carried a death sentence. Lesser violations of law were met with corporal punishments. Flogging was most popular since it was feared by the crew and didn't leave lasting damage if it was done within reasonable limits. A punished sailor was able to return to work after a short time to recover. The punishment could also be tailored to fit the crime. In cases of theft or pilfering, each crew member would deliver a lash with a small bit of rope to the offender as he was led past them. This was known as 'running the gauntlet'.

Originally, punishment could consist of hundreds of lashes, by the mid-1700's this was limited to a dozen due to the brutal nature of the cat-o-nine tails. The cat was made from thin lengths of waxed rope or cord. The ends were finished with knots known as blood knots, designed to bite into the skin. The cat was often referred to as the Captain's daughter.
Floggings were carried out in front of the crew as a deterrent to future crimes. When the flogging was done, the prisoner was taken below deck to have salt rubbed into the wounds. This served a dual purpose; to prevent infection and reinforce the punishment.

After flogging with the cat was banned, birching through clothing became an often used punishment for those under 18, while caning was used with adults. After the early 1900's, caning became the standard punishment for boys as well.

The ritual of punishment was designed to instill as much fear and discomfort as possible. The offender would be examined by a doctor then fitted with the thinnest possible cotton duck trousers. It is said that especially worn out trousers were kept on hand for the express purpose of punishment, to ensure that they didn't soften the blows.

Once properly dressed, the accused would stand and listen to the charges against him. The offence was read aloud, slowly, along with the punishment he was about to receive. He would then be held or tied in a bent over position, to expose the buttocks and pulling the threadbare trousers taut across the skin. It was called kissing the gunner's daughter since they were often bent over a field gun. Each stroke of the cane was delivered in a deliberate and precise way, often with pauses of up to a minute between each one. This served to draw out the punishment and ensure that the offender felt and remembered each blow.

Welts and bruises from caning could last up to 14 days. Care was taken to prevent infection if the skin was broken. Boys would often be allowed to eat meals while standing for a day or two after being punished.

Sometimes humiliation is a better deterrent than physical pain, although many punishments expertly combined both elements for maximum effect. We see this combination in the creative punishments of the US.

Bucking and gagging were popular for minor offences during the American civil war. The offender would be sat down with hands tied underneath legs and ankles tied together. This forced him into a bent forward position. A wooden dowel or stick would be placed in the mouth, like the bit of a horse.

Riding the wooden mule also appeared during the US civil war. It consisted of sitting astride a narrow board just high enough so that the feet couldn't touch the ground. There are even stories of buckets of water or sand being tied to the ankles of the accused to add to the discomfort.

English School Discipline

The cane is probably the most well-known implement of discipline in the English School system. Outlawed in British government schools in 1986 and not until 1998 in private schools (2000 for Scotland and 2003 for Northern Ireland!), caning was used widely in many schools. Due to the British Empire's influence on the world, their methods of punishment and discipline spread throughout the world. Some of the corporal punishments are still used today in parts of the world.

Traditionally, the cane (as well as the birch and other disciple methods) were applied to the buttocks or the palms of the hands. Cane strokes on the buttocks could be delivered with trousers on, for younger students, or on bare bottoms, generally for older students.

Canes were made from rattan, a strong, thick grass. It would be oiled to maintain flexibility. Soaked rattan (which makes it heavier and more flexible) is only used in judicial punishments in a few countries, due to its brutality. Canes could have a curved handle that resembles a shepherd's crook or ornately carved wooden handles. Some would have no handle at all.

In some schools, punishments were the sole domain of the Headmaster or Headmistress. In others, older students known as prefects were able to administer discipline for minor offences. As would be expected, this setup was ripe for abuse and was slowly phased out of most schools by the 1960's.

Birching, which caning replaced since it can be administered over clothing, was well used in British schools. A birch rod consists of many twigs bundled together, often from the birch tree - hence the name. The leaves and small twigs would be removed and the bundle would be held together by a cord or ribbon.

The positioning and procedure of caning and birching are very similar. Birching needed to be applied to the bare skin to be effective, while caning can be applied through clothing.

The offender would be bent over and may or may not have trousers removed. A birching horse was often employed, a saw horse style contraption with padding on the top, tall enough that the offender's feet are off the ground when in use. In modern BDSM dungeons, you will see many similar pieces of furniture, often referred to as a spanking horse or spanking bench. The person being punished can be bound to the birching horse if needed.

Generally, positioning involved having the legs together, to avoid hitting the back of the genitals, especially if the punishment is delivered without trousers.

Slippering was also popular in British homes and schools. This involved striking the palms of the hands or buttocks with a slipper. While this may sound mild compared to caning and birching, the 'slippers' generally employed were actually called a plimsoll or gym shoe. They had a heavy rubber sole that could impart quite a thud.

Slippering consisted of a few quick smacks on the buttocks while the student was bent over the teacher's desk. Sometimes it was done with the offender bent over grasping the thighs or touching toes, a position that is hard to maintain while being punished.

Ritual Pain

While many forms of ritual pain are used to show devotion to a god or gods, some religious practices involve causing pain as a form of self-discipline, to purge the body of sin.

This practice is most often observed in the Americas in the context of Catholicism, although it has roots in the Great Schism of 1054. It is after this time that the practice of mortification of the flesh became widespread. It was believed that suffering through physical trials or denying oneself comforts that the sinful nature present in every person could be 'put to death'.

Fasting, abstinence, and refraining from alcohol for a time were common ways to achieve this state and are still practised by mainstream Catholics today. Other methods included kneeling in prayer for hours, vows of poverty taken by monks, wearing a cilice (hairshirt) and self-flagellation with a discipline.

A cilice is an article of clothing that is woven out of coarse material or animal hair, giving it a very rough texture. Wearing it directly against the skin provides discomfort in penance for adorning oneself, so many famous figures in history have been known to wear them, including Charlemagne, Henry IV, Ivan the Terrible and Mother Teresa.

A discipline is a small bundle of knotted leather thongs. It was used as part of prayer, in a ritual of self-flagellation.

Many of the more extreme methods of attaining purity have fallen out of fashion in the past thousand years, however, some are still seen today in the developing world. Catholic self-flagellation is still commonly seen in Easter rituals throughout Latin America.

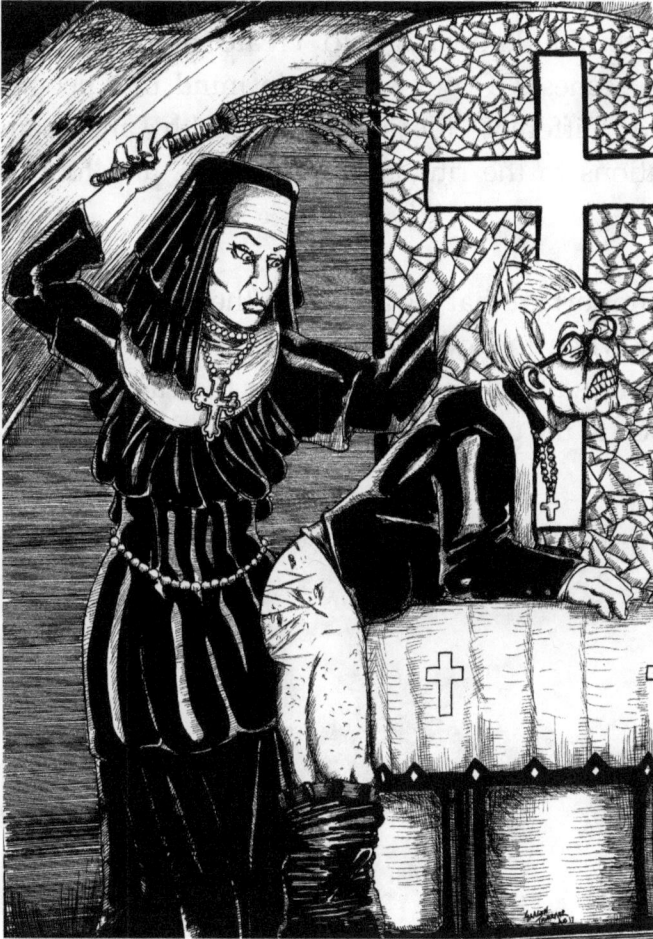

In addition to Catholicism, acts of self-flagellation can be seen in Islam, most notably in Shia communities, who engage in similar rituals during the Day of Ashura or Day of Atonement. Most commonly, devotees hit themselves in the chest during parades commemorating the death of Husayn ibn Ali. Some engage in the banned practice of striking themselves on the back with chains and knives.

Drawing Inspiration

History is a wonderful tool to use to draw inspiration for our scenes. If one area of history draws your attention, learn about it and use the knowledge to create more authentic and powerful scenes. Of course, keep in mind that people of the past had different ideas about health and safety, so modifications to the rituals, punishments, and tools may be needed.

It is also important that we approach these ideas with respect, especially when engaging in religious play. Some things may be better suited for private play rather than a fetish party that's open to the general public. Use your discretion and play safe!

Consent

Consent is key in BDSM. It is what separates kink from abuse and is essential for healthy BDSM relationships. There are different models of consent, but in most BDSM circles, affirmative consent is the baseline model.

Affirmative consent & Opt-in Negotiation

Affirmative consent states that in order to consent, a person must know what they are consenting to, including any reasonable risks or other adverse consequences. They must not be coerced or pressured into consenting in any way. They must not be under the influence or be in an altered state of mind. they must voluntarily and freely consent, and retain the ability to withdraw consent at any time.

Affirmative consent is generally an 'opt-in' system, where any activity not discussed and explicitly consented to is off the table. So if a Top comes up with a brilliant idea mid-scene, that the bottom hasn't consented to, the Top should not follow through with the idea until both are able to sit down and discuss it.

Mid-scene negotiation is frowned upon by many people. The bottom may be in 'subspace' and therefore altered and unable to provide proper consent. Some people become very compliant while they are playing and there are unscrupulous Tops that take advantage of this. The best way to avoid accidentally violating a person's consent is to not try to re-negotiate a scene part way through.

In planned BDSM scenes, the negotiation may happen hours or days (or more) ahead of time. Tops can keep a sense of mystery by giving a list of activities to the bottom and finding out which they consent to. The Top can then pick and choose from the list, surprising the bottom while still engaging in affirmative consent.

If your negotiations have happened in advance, you may want to check in before your scene to make sure that nothing has changed.

In pick-up style play - where people decide to play on a more spur of the moment way - the same type of negotiations can happen. At a party, a Top may open their toy bag and ask if there is anything that the bottom does not want to be used on them. They can negotiate the details of the play based on their mutual likes and the rules of the party (if applicable).

Opt-out negotiation

Another negotiation style that is popular in relationships is the opt-out style of negotiation. The people involved can decide what activities they do not want to engage in, leaving the rest 'on the table'.

While this type of negotiation is rather popular in BDSM, it does leave some things wide open - for instance, if the bottom didn't think of something that they don't want to agree to, and the Top didn't list it as a possibility, mistakes can happen. The

Top may think that they are okay to move forward with an activity, while the bottom is unhappy with it. Safe words can stop an activity, but the damage may already be done.

If you choose to use this style of negotiation, be aware of its limitations and prepared to accept the consequences.

Consensual non-consent

Consensual non-consent is generally a relationship style, where the Top/Dominant is able to do what they like - within negotiated boundaries, and the bottom must comply. These types of relationships involve a great deal of trust and generally are something that more dedicated couples (or more) agree to.

CNC and punishment dynamics have a fair bit in common, with some people regarding them as the same thing. In this scenario, the bottom would agree to a set of rules and the consequences that the Top deems fit. They may know the consequences ahead of time or they may be decided in a 'punishment fits the crime' style arrangement.

CNC has also been used to describe 'forced' scenes, such as rape play, by some in the kink community. This definition can cause confusion when CNC dynamics are mistaken for resistance play, so always make sure that everyone is on the same page when negotiating.

Safe words

Safe words are a way for Tops and bottoms to communicate while still being able to use words like 'no', 'stop', etc. in a scene. Many people enjoy the idea of 'forced' play and want to be able to indulge in the fantasy by the bottom saying 'no' and having the Top continue. This style of play is often referred to as 'resistance play'. The safe word allows for them to do this, while still having a word that actually means 'no' or 'stop'.

Common safe words are 'yellow' and 'red' or 'safe word'.These safe words are often in place at play parties and dungeons, so that there are standard words that everyone understands to mean 'no'. Yellow often means that a person is getting close to their limit of pain tolerance or their ability to handle the play. Red can mean either stop the scene entirely, or stop what is happening and check in.

The exact meaning of safe words must be negotiated between players so that there aren't any miscommunications.

Many people prefer to play in a way where regular language is used to communicate. This is a very common thing but should be discussed prior to play, so that everyone is on the same page.

Of course, safe words aren't magical and can not stop someone who is intent on violating consent. They are simply a communication tool for people to use (or not use) during BDSM play.

Special Considerations

There are some things that you should negotiate and get consent for specifically, especially if you are using an opt-out style of negotiation. These things can include sexual activity (which can include things such as STI status, safer sex practices, etc), leaving marks (including where marks are/not acceptable) and kink activities which are likely to trigger negative reactions in a large number of people, like face slapping. Edge play or riskier activities that involve breath play or blood should also be specifically discussed.

Punishment versus Funishment

Punishment is a common theme in a lot of BDSM play - even the "D" in the acronym can stand for discipline. Of course, like everything else in BDSM, this isn't as straightforward as one might expect. Many people have different ideas of what punishment entails.

Punishment is generally accepted to be the consequence for poor behaviour, including the imposition of a penalty against the person in the wrong. This penalty can be any number of things. In BDSM it commonly takes the form of privileges revoked, acts of contrition or corporal punishments.

Of course, not all relationships include a punishment dynamic. Many BDSM practitioners, whether into bedroom only kink or full-time D/s relationships, have little interest in actual punishment. They prefer to talk about transgressions, create strategies to prevent future offences or end the relationship (if the transgression is severe enough).

At the same time, many people eroticise punishment.

In order to describe this situation, where people enjoy the idea of punishment, but who also don't want to break the rules of their relationship agreements, we use the term "funishment".

Funishment is the sort of "you've been very, very bad; now I'm going to spank you (wink, wink, nudge, nudge)". It's a way of playing with the concept of punishment without anyone getting hurt in ways they don't want to be.

Funishments can be given for anything - whether it actually happened or not. I've been known to 'funish' bottoms because

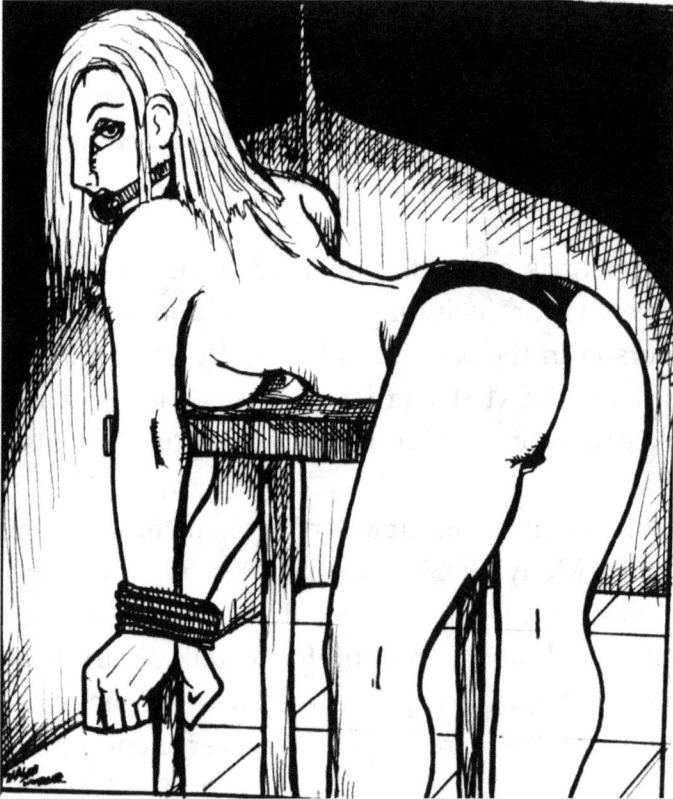

of things which may or may not have happened - I just needed an excuse! The great thing about this type of play is that it does involve a bit of role-playing, so you can feel free to make things up as you go along. We will go into more detail later on in "Building a Scene".

When negotiating your relationship or any BDSM play, it is important to make this distinction - whether you chose to use the term funishment or not. Personally, I am not interested in a partner who breaks rules to invoke punishment. I would not last long in a relationship where this was going on. I do enjoy a partner who can express, in words, that they would like to play. I also don't mind a partner who will be 'bratty' to encourage funishment, although I can be very picky about this behaviour, a common thing among Dominants of all stripes.

Guidelines for negotiating punishment dynamics will be discussed in a later chapter, here we will focus more on how to play with funishment.

In general, it is unwise to use funishment in regards to actual transgressions. Think about it, if your partner is aroused by or enjoys 'punishments' you are encouraging rule breaking. Essentially, you are rewarding bad behaviour, by giving them something they enjoy when they have broken an agreed upon rule.

If you are not engaging in a PE relationship, you likely will not have rules governing your partner's behaviour. If this is the case, a set of play or fun rules may be ideal. Your partner can break them without worrying about genuinely upsetting you and you have an excuse to 'punish' them. As long as you're both on the same page, this can work out quite well.

Example of Play/Fun Rules List
(Rules for Play Time or Parties)

1. Bottom will thank Top after each strike during play
2. Bottom will count each strike during play
3. Bottom will thank Top for any corrections to behaviour
4. Bottom will not make eye contact with Top
5. Bottom will not speak without permission from Top
6. Bottom will not sit on furniture, either standing behind/beside Top, or kneeling/sitting on the floor
7. Bottom will use an honorific for Top
8. Bottom will serve Top food and drink, presenting it by kneeling in front of Top and waiting to be acknowledged
9. Bottom will ensure that Top is comfortable at all times, providing foot rubs, massages, drinks, or another service when requested
10. Bottom will dress (or undress, as appropriate) to please Top

If you decide to use these rules, or ones you make up yourself, you can see how there would be lots of ways for a bottom to rack up funishments. The bottom can easily 'forget' to use the appropriate honorific or *gasp* sit on the furniture. Neither of these things would be hurtful to the Top, but it is a way for the bottom to create a reason to play.

During play, the bottom can rack up further funishment, by breaking further rules. They could 'forget' what number they're on, 'forget' to say thank you, etc. While some people may feel like this is topping from the bottom, or giving the bottom too much control over play, others will find it a fun way to communicate without getting out of the punishment headspace.

Now, if you are engaging in a PE relationship, you may already have a set of rules that you and your partner must follow. In this case, you could decide to have two sets of rules, your real rules that shouldn't be broken and a set of rules that you don't care about, that your partner can break to indicate that they are wanting play. I am not a fan of this approach because lines can become blurry and it makes me feel as if I'm performing for my partner, instead of leading our relationship. However, if you don't feel the same way, this can be a fun, albeit complicated, method.

Despite this, specific play rules can still work, such as the ones regarding counting strikes or saying thank you after each one. While I don't implement these types of rules every time (as a sadist, the unending counting would get on my nerves), I do use them sometimes if I want to allow my partner a bit of control during play time.

If you chose to take this approach, it is very important to be clear about which rules are just for fun. If you are taking a rule seriously and your partner isn't, you may end up feeling disobeyed if you are the Dominant/Top or you may not understand what is expected of you, if you are the submissive/bottom. Generally, it's best to implement these play rules after you have an established dynamic, so that there is less confusion.

Physical Safety & Anatomy for BDSM

It is a well-known adage in the BDSM world that you want to avoid striking the lower back of a person, due to the potential for damage to their kidneys. How true is this? Where is it safe to strike a person? How hard? With which implements? In this chapter, we will answer these questions, so that you can feel comfortable and confident in your discipline sessions as well as in general BDSM play.

The body provides many wonderful places to land a blow and a few you should avoid. Generally speaking, striking any well-muscled part of the body is relatively safe. Hitting the joints or unprotected organs can cause problems. Let's start at the top of the head and work our way down, discussing the places where you should and shouldn't strike.

I should also make clear that while I have worked in the healthcare field in the past, I am not a doctor and my advice here should not replace the advice of a doctor. If you have any questions regarding your ability to engage in kink play, many doctors are open minded and understand that some people choose to engage in consensual BDSM. If you are embarrassed asking about kink, ask about your fitness to engage in 'contact sports' such as martial arts.

Keep in mind that there is no truly safe way to hit or play, as everything carries risks. By becoming informed, you can determine your own risk tolerance and make informed choices when it comes to BDSM.

Head and Neck

The head itself is a bit of a no-go zone. You don't want to strike the top or back of the head because you could potentially do damage, but more likely you will give your bottom a headache. There is very little padding between the skin and the bone, which means any blows will just hurt in an unpleasant way. Hard blows or striking with implements have the potential to cut skin, cause concussions or worse. It's best to avoid striking the top or back of the head.

Striking the face can be done, but it takes a good deal of precision and should really only be done with open hands - no implements. It is also important to support the head by holding the other side of the face to avoid sudden head and neck movements. Face slapping can be fun, but a misplaced strike can cause damage to the orbital bone, nose or jaw. Striking the ear, on purpose or by accident, has the potential to damage the eardrum and the cartilage in the ear. Forcing air into the ear canal through a strike can rupture or otherwise damage the eardrum. Have you seen the 'cauliflower ears' that some boxers get? It's from multiple strikes damaging the cartilage of the ear, resulting in scar tissue building up. While ears are fun to grab and twist, they shouldn't be hit.

The neck is off limits. Striking any part of the neck has the potential for serious consequences. Damage can be done to the spine by harder blows to the back of the neck, with the potential for pinched nerves, swelling, pain, and damage to the bones of the neck. Striking the front of the neck can cause damage to the trachea and/or larynx, which can have potentially serious results. While some people enjoy breath play and blood chokes, that type of play carries high risks and is beyond the purview of this book, so will not be discussed.

Joints

The joints of the shoulder, elbow, wrist, knee and ankle are considered no-go zones for most types of BDSM play. Impact should not be used on the joints at all since it is fairly easy to cause damage. Bondage should avoid most joints, although properly applied bondage over the wrists and ankles is OK

The reason that joints are best avoided is two-fold. There are mechanical considerations - joints are less stable than a part of the body and can be dislocated or damaged if enough force is applied. The other reason is that arteries, veins, and nerves are much closer to the surface at the joints and have very little protection. Damage to these structures can cause a myriad of problems, including excessive bleeding, pain, and loss of movement/sensation.

Chest

Looking at the front of the body, we come to the chest. There will be some variation on risks depending on how much breast tissue is present. Typically, men will have very little breast tissue, whereas women will have a greater amount. People who have had mastectomies may have had some or all of the breast tissue excised. Breast implants carry their own risks when it comes to play.

Causing trauma to the breasts or chest by impact or other means can cause micro-bleeds; tiny amounts of bleeding in the breast tissue. As these injuries heal, they can become calcified. Small calcifications can confuse radiologists when looking at a mammogram if they are unaware of the patient's history of trauma or BDSM activities. The calcifications, if there are a lot of them, can also obscure actual tumours The result can be unneeded tests and biopsies or in a worst case scenario, a missed or late diagnosis of cancer.

Repeated trauma can also cause the tissues to harden, whether or not there is breast tissue present. This does take a long time to occur and is more frequently seen in other parts of the body - leather butt is a fairly well-known complication of regular play on the ass, but it can happen to the breasts/chest as well.

While unlikely, repeated trauma to the skin, chronic inflammation and the presence of scars can result in a Marjolin's ulcer. These are a form of cancer, which is quite aggressive. Generally, they form on skin with frequent wounds and can take many years to form. Again, these ulcers can form on any part of the body, not just the chest.

Fat necrosis is another risk from heavy impact and trauma to the breasts/chest. It can present as a lump that the person finds themselves or can be detected during routine medical screening and can be mistaken for a cancerous tumour

With that said, impact on the breasts/chest is a low to medium risk form of play, depending on how hard the play is and what types of implements are used.

Surface-oriented impact (stingy toys, generally), will help to reduce the risk of calcifications and fat necrosis in breasts. Lighter impact can also help with this.

Breast/chest bondage can also present some risks. Be aware that tight bondage around the chest can interfere with the ability to take a deep breath or to breathe properly. Bottoms in tight bondage which includes the chest should be monitored closely for breathing issues, which may become worse over time.

Compression of the breasts causes vascular constriction. This is particularly important when it comes to breast tissue because of the greater presence of endocrine tissue which carries lymphatic fluid. This fluid is part of the immune system and plays a major role in destroying abnormal cells. Many Tops choose to limit the time that breasts are bound because of this.

It should also be noted that nipples are erectile tissue, not breast tissue, so can be compressed (nipple clamps, etc) for short periods of time without the same risks.

Finally, breast implants should be treated with care. Heavy impact can damage the implant, depending on its placement. Tight breast bondage should not be considered, as it can place too much pressure on an implant and cause a rupture. As always, the advice of your surgeon should always be heeded.

Arms

Arms are a fairly safe area to play, with the exception of the joints of the elbow and wrist. The underarm (armpit) should be avoided for most types of play as well; it's the underside of the shoulder joint and the skin can be delicate. While tickling is OK, impact or bondage is not.

The upper arms are fairly tough. Be aware that the radial nerve can be close to the surface, generally on the outside or back of the arm, a little higher than halfway between the shoulder and the elbow. Compression or trauma to the nerve can cause sensory defects and loss of movement.

The forearms are also alright for play, as long as heavy impact is avoided.

Hands

The hands contain many small bones which can be easily broken by hard impact. If you choose to play with the hands, you should avoid the top. The palm and underside of the fingers are OK for light or stingy impact, but proceed with caution - it's easy to cause injury accidentally. The skin of the back of the hand can be fairly stretchy, but it also tends to be delicate. Be careful and start slow/light when incorporating hands into your play.

Stomach

While the stomach area is fine for some types of play, it is not appropriate for impact play. Don't believe everything you see in the movies, flogging the stomach is neither sexy or fun for most bottoms!

The stomach area is where you will find many internal organs, including the stomach itself, the kidneys, liver, and intestines. The rib cage offers some protection for the sides, but very little in the front. While bottoms will have varying degrees of muscle to protect the organs, it is unwise to do heavy impact play in this area. If you want to engage in impact play over the stomach, stick to stingy implements that are surface oriented. Martial artists and other fighters are trained in how to receive a blow to the stomach, many bottoms aren't.

Genitals

Genitorture is a very popular form of BDSM play. It is, however, beyond the purview of this book so will not be discussed in detail.

Vulvae are pretty resilient and can handle most forms of impact play as well as a wide variety of other types of play. Penises and scrotum's can also handle a surprising amount of impact, with a few caveats. Be careful not to apply too much force to a single testicle as you can cause a rupture. Twisting of the scrotum should be avoided at all costs since it can cause a testicular torsion - a situation which requires immediate emergency medical care.

If you do want to include genital play, start light and go slow. Also highly recommend learning specific techniques, either through in-person education, books or online instruction.

Hips

The hip area should generally be avoided when it comes to impact play. The area is not well muscled and may not have a lot of fat covering it. The bones are close to the surface as is the sciatic nerve.

The sciatic nerve runs from the spine, through the hips, and down each leg. Impact to the hips can cause inflammation which can, in turn, compress the nerve. The nerve can also become pinched at the joint. These things can cause a large degree of pain and make walking difficult. The pain can last for hours, days, weeks or more.

As with other joints, it's best to avoid play in the hip area.

Thighs (front & inside)

The front of the thighs is very resilient. They are heavily muscled and have a layer of fat covering them. Impact play is fine in this area, provided your aim is good. It can be very easy to 'wrap' implements because of the shape of the leg. Be aware that any flexible implement is capable of wrapping, which can be painful and even dangerous at times.

This part of the body is also not used to impact. It will generally bruise more readily than the buttocks. If you want to avoid bruises, a good warm up and lighter play may be in order.

The inside of the thighs are also fine for play, but they are much more sensitive. They're a generally protected area, so will bruise very easily. Be aware that play and joints don't mix, so stay away from the area where the leg meets the torso.

Shins

While light play is okay in this area, there is no muscle to protect the bone. This also means that the skin is more likely to break when hit. Shins should be left for sensation play or very light impact play (but there are so many other, better parts of the body to hit, you probably shouldn't bother).

Feet

Like the hands, the feet have many small bones that can be easily damaged. Foot torture can be a lot of fun if you know what you're doing. Impact play should be kept to the bottoms of the feet and require good aim. Again, being well versed in the appropriate technique is key to a safe foot torture session.

Calves

The back of the lower leg, where the calf muscle is located, is fine for impact play. Just be aware of the knee joint above and the ankle joint below. You want to stick to the area of the muscle, otherwise, you run into the same problems as the shin. In addition, there are a number of tendons, nerves and blood vessels close to the surface near the ankle that should not be hit. Be careful of wrapping in this area as well.

Hamstrings

The back of the upper legs is a great place for impact play. They are more sensitive than the buttocks, so Tops should keep that in mind. They are heavily muscled and often have a thick layer of fat covering them. Be aware that it is easy to wrap flexible implements around the leg and hit the hip, which will be more painful than intended and can possibly break the skin. It can also be easy to accidentally hit the genitals, depending on the position of the legs. Observe caution in this area to ensure that you only hit the genitals when you want to, not because of poor aim.

Buttocks

The buttocks are easily the most popular site for impact play and are well suited for it. The area is protected by large muscles, generally, has a good layer of fat for additional protection and any nerves or blood vessels are away from the surface. Additionally, the bottom can bend over and be in a stable position, sometimes with the help of dungeon furniture, for play.

Leather butt, as mentioned in the section on breasts, is a well-known occurrence in the kink world. The repeated use of impact on the buttocks can cause the skin to toughen up and become like leather. The skin becomes less sensitive, requiring more force to get a reaction from the bottom. Calcifications can also occur, toughening the tissue under the skin.

Extended or heavy impact scenes can also cause inflammation, which can cause nerves to be compressed. If symptoms of sciatica or other nerve compression are associated with heavy impact play on the buttocks, it is best to take some time off to let everything heal (you can still play on different parts of the body).

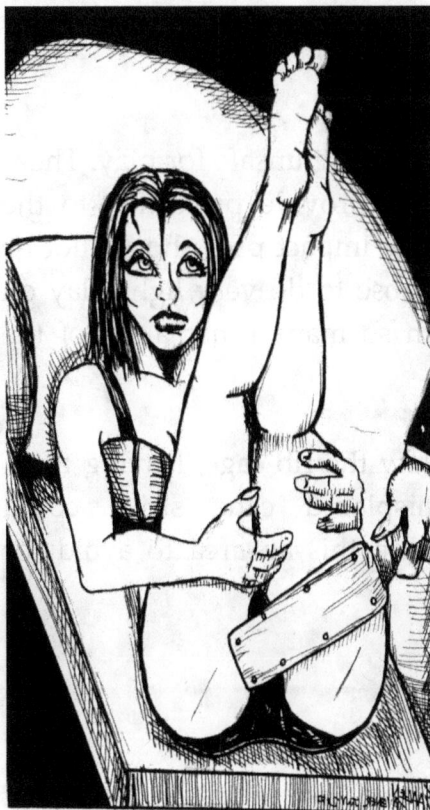

Heavy impact can also cause scar tissue to form, which can add to the desensitization of the buttocks. Massage has been shown to help break up scar tissue, the addition of lotions is optional. You may want to incorporate some massage into your aftercare routine for heavy play, techniques for breaking up scar tissue can be found online.

Tops should also be aware that hitting the tailbone can cause pain and injury to the bottom. If your aim isn't 100% accurate, be sure to place something over the tailbone to protect it while playing.

The 'sweet spot'

The small crease where the back of the legs meets the buttocks is known as the 'sweet spot'. While it's quite sweet for Tops, it is less so for bottoms. It is a part of the buttocks that is more protected and more sensitive than the rest because it doesn't get toughened up by sitting or contact with other objects. A skilled Top will be able to place a cane strike in the sweet spot, hopefully getting a good reaction from the bottom. It can also be taken advantage of with spanking and many other types of play.

Lower Back

The lower back is well known for being unsafe for play. There is a lack of muscle and bone to provide protection to the internal organs, which means that impact play should not be considered. Some Tops may choose to do very light play on the lower back, but again, with so many other areas of the body, why bother?

The kidneys poke out from below the rib cage, leaving them vulnerable to impact. A misplaced cane strike could potentially cause damage, making this an area to avoid for most types of play.

Upper back

Next, to the buttocks, this is the most popular spot for impact play, especially flogging. With lots of muscle, the area can take a good deal of punishment.

Be aware that protruding shoulder blades, whether a result of positioning or a bottom without much muscle or fat, can become painful and cause the skin to break with some types of play. Try to position your bottom where their arms are relaxed at their sides or bound in such a way that their shoulder blades aren't protruding too much (like when they're tied to a St. Andrew's Cross).

It should also be noted that hitting the spine should be avoided at all times. Hitting the spine can cause direct damage and it can cause minor misalignment which can result in back pain. The spine is not protected by muscle and is more vulnerable to impact because of this. It is also easier to break skin unintentionally because of the lack of muscle over the bone.

Special Considerations

- Bruising may take a few hours to a few days to develop fully. Getting to know your partner's body is essential in only causing bruises that you intend to. Many factors play into the formation of a bruise, so 'no marks' can't really be guaranteed, even by the most skilled professional.
- Older people will bruise more easily than younger people. As we age, skin becomes thinner and less elastic, which leaves it more prone to being bruised.
- Fatty areas tend to bruise more easily than muscled areas. Women tend to have more subcutaneous fat, which means they bruise more easily.
- In areas where there is no padding between the skin and bone (so no muscle or fat), can be prone to having the skin break unintentionally. Be careful in these areas and understand which types of implements are more likely to cause accidental damage, such as canes (in this case).

Protecting the Body

While it is important to perfect your aim with an implement before using it, you may also want to take measures to protect various parts of the body, especially during heavy scenes. When striking a person with great intensity, precision can be lost. In these cases, it is often better to be safe, rather than sorry, by taking precautions.

When striking the upper back, a small mistake can result in an implement hitting the back of the neck or head. At best, this is an annoying thing for your bottom, at worst, it could cause injury. It is wise to have your bottom keep their head forward when you strike. Bottoms may arch their backs and put their heads back after an intense blow, so it is important to know how your bottom will react. You may need to give them some time to recover between blows and remind them to return to the position you require before continuing.

You can also place something over the back of their neck to help protect it from an errant blow. The bottom's shirt, a small folded throw blanket or anything similar can be enough to deflect or spread out a poorly aimed strike. Of course, if you find yourself striking this padding too often, you will want to stop and practice a lot more before attempting that play again.

If you are striking the chest and/or breasts of the bottom, a misplaced blow can easily hit their throat or face. Having them put their head back is wise, and you can use the same technique to protect the throat as you did with the back of the neck.

With a bottom bent over so that you can strike the buttocks, placing something over the tailbone and lower back can help protect it. It can also help if you are unsure of where you should be aiming. Using your hands, feel out where the bottom's tailbone is. You can then place their shirt, a folded towel or even a flogger over the tailbone area.

Again, if you find that you are hitting the padding frequently, you need to work on your aim. This should be a precaution for accidents, not a solution for a lack of aim.

You can even use this safety precaution as a bit of a game with your bottom. Tell them they must stay still and not drop or knock the item off their body. If they squirm too much and the padding falls, they will earn extra funishment.

If your bottom has a penis and scrotum that you have decided to torture, there are pieces of equipment that you can use to isolate the genitals away from the body. A trampling board, a half box that goes over the body that has a hole for the genitals to poke through can be used. You can then flog or hit the genitals without hitting the stomach (which probably wouldn't cause injury, but certainly won't feel good either).

Larger breasts can also be isolated from the rest of the body in much the same way that the penis and scrotum can be. A board or box with space for the breasts to protrude though can be an aid for play and feel objectifying for the bottom.

Using secure bondage can help cut down on struggling and squirming, keeping the bottom in the position you want them in and helping to avoid misplaced blows. By becoming proficient with rope, you can ensure that your bottom stays where you want them, no matter how strange the position. Other restraints are a great solution for those who aren't fans of rope (or just want to secure the bottom quickly). While they are more limited in scope, many bottoms enjoy the feel of leather or steel restraints.

Items like stocks/pillories and various types of dungeon furniture can also be used to secure your bottom. Stocks can be attached to a stand (pillory) or be used on their own. Ankle stocks are great for isolating the feet for bastinado, for example. Spreader bars can also be used in a similar way, to limit movement and position the bottom.

If you so desire, you can train your bottom to hold positions and not move. This is known as verbal or mental bondage. It can take a good deal of training and discipline to teach a bottom to stay still, even during intense sensations. A good deal of self-control is required on the part of the bottom and a good deal of patience is needed for the top, but verbal/mental bondage can be quite effective.

At the end of the day, the best way to protect your bottoms body is through practice with implements - each and every one, not just one of each type. Every individual implement is different. The use of one crop is the same as another, but there are variations between crops. One may be longer or shorter, more or less flexible, have a smaller or larger tress. Make sure that you are proficient with every implement in your collection, or don't use it. If you haven't used an implement in a while, or it's brand new, spend some time beating a pillow before looking at your bottom.

Remember, as a Top, it is your responsibility to care for the safety and well-being of your bottom during the scene. If you neglect this responsibility, you could injure your partner, a situation that no one wants.

Protecting the Mind

There is a good deal of attention paid to physical safety in BDSM, which is incredibly important, however, psychological safety can sometimes be overlooked. When we are engaging in activities like power exchange, punishment/funishment and consensual non-consent, we run the risk of psychological 'injury'. This isn't limited to the bottom, although they generally bear the brunt of the risks. Psychological safety is part of the motivation for aftercare in kinky practices, but it isn't the only thing we need to do.

I need to make it clear that I am not a psychologist. I am writing from my personal experience and research - both through medical literature and by talking to other BDSM practitioners. What I have written in this section (or any of the book) should not be taken as gospel, and it should never replace the advice or opinion of an actual doctor. If you or your partner(s) find yourselves in crisis, don't hesitate to ask for assistance from friends or mental health professionals.

There are some things which affect both Tops and bottoms, others are more specific to the role. Things like frenzy and drop can affect anyone, even though they are often associated with bottoms.

Frenzy is a reaction to discovering BDSM, after having fantasized about it for years. When a person finds that there is a whole community of people just like them, and all sorts of options to satisfy the urges they've tried to keep quiet, they can go a little overboard. It often looks like a person doing all sorts of play with all sorts of people, with little regard for personal safety or the consequences.

Of course, frenzy can hit anyone at anytime, even more, experienced kinksters. If you discover a type of play that's new to you that you really enjoy, you can end up in a frenzy, trying to do everything possible in a short period of time.

While I think it's a perfectly natural reaction to become a little obsessed with something that makes us happy, it can lead to problems. People can easily get in over their heads, often by doing play they don't have the skill for or by playing with people they normally wouldn't under normal circumstances. It is an obsession, putting the need to satisfy kink needs over other considerations.

In most circumstances, frenzy passes without issue. Sometimes it can cause more lasting problems; unintentionally hurting long-term partners in favour of the new and shiny things or people; unsafe play; taking risks that one normally wouldn't; partners who violate consent.

The best way to handle frenzy is to set limits for yourself. It can help to share with a friend you trust, who can give you honest advice on the choices you're making. Having feedback from a trusted source can help us see things that we may overlook, whether it's our own less than safe obsessions or spending time with the wrong sort of people.

Many people are familiar with the idea of 'sub-drop' but don't realize that there is also 'Top-drop'. Drop, in general, describes a feeling of sadness, emptiness or vulnerability after engaging in BDSM activities. This can happen within a few hours of play or even a few days later.

There is no science to tell us why this happens. Some believe that it's due to the release of endorphins during play. Endorphins make us feel good and when they're gone we can feel let down. Other explanations are more psychological, that the connections we make while playing are so intense that we feel lost without them.

I am not sure what the causes of drop are, only that it happens to many people. For some, it is predictable, they will feel drop after they play, every time. For others, it can be unpredictable; some scenes may leave them with drop, while others have no after-effects.

If you do experience drop, there are many ideas of how to deal with it. Many people find they need something sweet to eat after they play. Others just need to eat - I find that play leaves me very hungry! Some people find that cuddling and reconnecting with their partner helps with any negative feelings. Yet other people prefer to be left alone to process their feelings (physical or emotional). These activities, and much more, are referred to as aftercare. There are as many ways of dealing with drop as there are people who experience it. You may need to try a number of things before finding what works for you.

It is important to understand that drop is a common reaction to BDSM activities - on both sides of the slash. It is also important to know if you require aftercare and what you need. Both Tops and bottoms can need or want aftercare.

For Tops

Much of the focus on health and safety is directed at Tops as instructions on how to keep bottoms safe. This is incredibly important, and a serious responsibility that Tops take on. However, Tops also need to look after themselves. They run into different, but very legitimate, psychological issues when it comes to BDSM.

One of the most common issues that Tops run into when they first start playing (or if they decide to play harder, causing bruising, etc) is the "am I a monster?" question. This is especially prevalent with sadistic Tops - they pain they want to cause it at odds with their sense of self. We all like to believe that we are good people, and we are taught from a young age that good people don't hurt others.

This is closely tied in with the things we teach our young men (and people who are assigned male at birth - AMAB), that they should never hit women (cis, trans, or non-binary folks who sometimes present as women). These messages are ingrained in us as children and can be incredibly difficult to overcome.

While everyone is different and some people are never able to overcome this programming (or may not want to, preferring to be a 'sensual Top/Dominant'), it is important to remember that BDSM activities are happening with consent. Consent is what separates what we do from abuse. Some people do prefer to negotiate in a different way, but the general standard for consent is the 'affirmative consent' model. This helps re-assure the Top that the bottom is a willing participant. By giving consent to specific activities, the bottom can let the top know that they are wanting to participate in the activities, either for their own enjoyment or because a punishment dynamic suits them best in a relationship.

Consent is also what separates BDSM from domestic abuse. The other key point here is that punishments should not be doled out in anger in a punishment dynamic. This will be discussed in more detail later on, but genuine punishments should be discussed between the people involved before being carried out.

It is not uncommon to find that as the connection between Top and bottom becomes more intense, that the Top has a hard time in punishing the bottom (or engaging in funishment style play). This is especially noticeable in romantic relationships, where the partners fall in love. Many Tops forget that their bottoms may be masochists or otherwise crave BDSM play, and begin to fall into the 'am I a monster?' trap above.

Masochistic bottoms crave physical or emotional pain. It gets them off, it makes them happy, it makes them feel whole - or they may have entirely different reasons for enjoying pain. Chances are, they will not be satisfied in a relationship where some sort of consensual pain is not present.

A phrase that I often find myself saying is "Pain is Sadist for 'I love you'." My partners are always masochists of some sort, and submissive. I know what I need and want in a relationship, and because I've done that soul-searching, I am able to look for partners who are appropriate for me. Because I know that my partners crave my love and affection in a way that is complementary to the way I express it (masochism to my sadism), I don't have to worry about feeling like a monster or a bad person for wanting to cause my partner pain.

For Bottoms

Just like Tops can feel like monsters for wanting to cause pain, bottoms can feel 'less than' for wanting to receive pain. This can manifest in a few different ways, and gender can often play a role.

Women (cis, trans or non-binary folks who sometimes present as women) often identify as feminists but run into a disconnect when they desire to bottom or submit to men (cis, trans or non-binary folks who sometimes present as men). While these feelings are often stronger in cis women submitting to cis men, they can be an issue for people across the gender spectrum.

There is a feeling that one can not be a 'good feminist' and have a desire to submit to a man (and male Tops can also feel that they aren't good feminists or allies by being dominant to a woman). It is important to remember that modern, intersectional feminism fights to allow all people to live their lives in the way that makes them happy, regardless of gender identity or kink orientation (to name a few things). If you are a woman (of any description) who enjoys submitting to a man (of any description), modern feminists should support your choice, because it is your choice. While I'm sure some more radical feminists may not like what you're doing, but you are free to live your life in the way you want, doing what makes you happy. If being a submissive feminist is what you want, then it is an identity that should be respected.

In the same vein, many men, often cis men, but sometimes trans men and non-binary people, find that there are negative stereotypes around them submitting or bottoming. While this is the expected role that women play in a patriarchal system, men are expected to be strong and in charge - not bottoming or submitting, especially to a woman identified person. Submission and bottoming are seen as weak, or less than.

In the same way that women identified people should be free to make the choices that make them happy, so should people who identify as men. Submission and bottoming are not signs of weakness, physical or mental. There is great strength and self-knowledge in being able to submit or bottom, especially when it goes against social norms.

Bottoms and submissives have generally done a bit of soul-searching, learning about themselves and their desires. In knowing that this is what they want and crave, whether in a relationship or just for fun, they have shown strength, not weakness.

There are many other psychological pitfalls that both Tops and bottoms, Dominants and submissives can fall into, but these are the most common for those both new and experienced in BDSM. If you find yourself worried about any of these issues, remember that you are not alone in feeling this way. The best way to help overcome these types of feelings is to talk to both your partner and to others with a similar identity.

Of course, switches can experience any of these issues and may experience some that are more specific to Tops and others that are more specific to bottoms. They may also find that they are more easily able to overcome them, by being able to experience the other side of the slash. Switches may even find that they experience other issues, not listed here, that are unique to being a switch.

The Positions of Punishment

Positioning can play an important role in punishment or funishment scenes. Not only can it add to the headspace of the person being punished but it can make actions more or less intense. By being aware of some basic positions and the effect they have, you will be better able to make use of positioning in your play or punishment scenes.

Over the Knee

Over the knee (OTK) is a popular position for spanking. It can be modified to be more or less strenuous or adapted for people with less mobility or strength. The basic position involves having the bottom bent over the knee of the Top.

When the Top is sitting on a chair, the bottom should be stretched across their lap, with both hands and feet on the ground (if they can reach). This way, the bottom can help support themselves in the case of a smaller Top and larger bottom. If the bottom can not reach the ground with both hands and feet, they should be able to reach with at least their hands or feet to help support themselves if needed.

If this positioning doesn't work for either the Top or the bottom, because of mobility issues, weight or any other reason, you can try having the bottom laying across the lap of the Top. The Top should be seated on a couch or the edge of a bed. The bottom will then lay across the Top's lap, with most of their weight supported by the furniture. Again, if you need to relieve more weight, the bottom can prop themselves up with elbows and thighs or knees.

When the Top is seated on a chair, they can exercise more control over the bottom by holding the bottom in place with a leg. Take the leg closest to the bottom's legs and put it over top. This will help prevent the bottom from squirming too much. This is generally easier to do when the Top is physically larger than the bottom, but it is possible even with a smaller Top.

This position presents the buttocks nicely for the Top to spank. OTK also provides great access to the 'sweet spot' so that a Top can take full advantage of this sensitive area. It is perfect when doing hand spankings or using other short implements. It is difficult to use longer implements due to the close proximity of both partners - there isn't enough room to swing a flogger, for instance.

The bottom can feel unbalanced in this position, which can be both a good and a bad thing. It is good if the Top wants to keep the bottom on their toes (quite literally). It can be bad if the physical uncertainty of the position takes away from focusing on the sensation of being spanked.

In this position, the skin and muscles are stretched a small amount, which will add a small bit of intensity to what the Top is doing. This intensity can be adjusted by how far the bottom is bent over, the further the bend, the more intense impact will feel.

This position often evokes memories of childhood punishment and is an iconic image within BDSM. It is a perfect choice when doing scenes that involve domestic discipline, or any scene where the bottom takes on a more childlike head space.

Laying flat

Laying flat and face down on a bed, bench or any other surface can give a Top many options for play or punishment. This is an ideal position for hard caning sensual play; it is very diverse. This position can be combined with bondage, such as rope or cuffs, or the Top can simply order the bottom to lay down. Some Tops may even enjoy using their bodies to restrain the bottom, by sitting on them.

This position is often the most comfortable for a bottom, although some may have a hard time laying face down. You can add a pillow under the hips to eliminate back arching and it has the added bonus of presenting the buttocks a bit. By using a pillow, you get a position that's part way between laying flat and OTK. Tops also have the option to tell the bottom to roll over, so that the Top has access to the chest/breast area, upper legs, and genitals.

Depending on whether or not you use bondage, and how tight the restraint is, the bottom can have a lot or very little wiggle room. This can be adjusted through the scene, perhaps restricting movement as things become more intense (or allowing the bottom more freedom to move during intense scenes so that they can process sensation better).

This position will not add any intensity to what the Top is doing. With the bottom laying comfortably on their stomach, the muscles of the buttocks are relaxed and the skin is not stretched at all. In this way, the bottom may be able to handle sensations that they wouldn't be able to take in a position that makes things feel more intense.

Standing

While it may seem obvious, spankings and other punishments/funishments can be delivered to a standing bottom. This is convenient for people who don't have extensive BDSM furniture or those who enjoy the concept of mental bondage (where the Top/Dominant commands the bottom/submissive to hold a position and not move).

While simply standing may not seem like the most exciting position, it can be made more interesting by having the bottom stand with their hands behind their head or folded behind their back. Legs can be together or spread apart. If you want parts of the bottom lower, have them kneel.

You can also add to the intensity of the position by making the surface uncomfortable. Having a bottom stand in bare feet on bamboo mat (the type made of actual bamboo twigs, not the flat kind), gravel, fake turf or other uncomfortable surfaces can make a scene more intense and interesting. Kneeling in uncooked rice on a hard surface is a classic punishment method.

You can also employ bondage with standing if you wish. You can have the bottom's hands bound above their head and attached to an overhead point (the use of suspension cuffs and a secure point is wise, in case the bottom faints). For shorter bottoms, you can even use an over the door towel hook to secure the bondage. Of course, if you have access, a whipping post or frame is a traditional punishment option and a St. Andrew's Cross is a staple in most dungeons. Many classic whipping frames look much like a ladder propped up at an angle, something that should be relatively easy to make for those so inclined.

Bent over object

This position puts the bottom in a similar position to the OTK position but will allow the Top more movement and the ability to use a variety of implements.

Bottoms can be bent over any solid object that you happen to have. Make sure that the object will not move or tip over with the weight of the bottom. Spanking horses and benches are popular dungeon furniture for this position. At home, you can bend a bottom over a counter, couch, bed or table; as long as the object is solid enough to hold the bottom's weight without moving.

Bondage can be used to secure the bottom or they can be left free to hold a position on their own. This position can be effective for heavier play, giving the bottom something to lean against, so they can focus on processing sensation rather than staying upright.

By bending over, usually at a 90-degree angle, the muscles and skin of the buttocks are stretched and adds intensity to the sensations the Top is giving. It is important to keep in mind what positioning does to intensity so that you can adjust as needed, perhaps with a longer warm up or less intense toys.

Touching Toes

Touching the toes is a fairly intense spanking position that may not be possible for all bottoms, due to a lack of flexibility or balance.

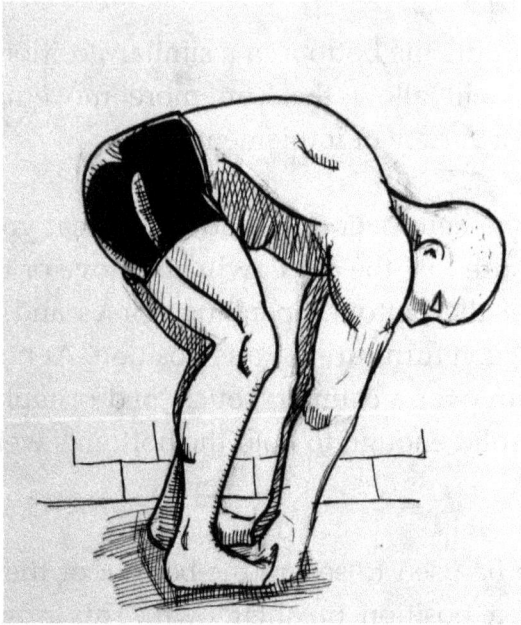

The bottom should stand, bending at the hips and reaching to touch the toes with the hands. Feet can be kept together if the bottom is flexible and stable enough in that position, or legs may be adjusted so that the feet are around shoulder width apart for more stability.

Many bottoms will not be flexible enough to reach their toes but bending at the hips with hands resting on the thighs or knees is also acceptable. Most important here is that the bottom can maintain their balance and not fall over. Bondage is not recommended for this position for this reason.

Due to the strenuous nature of the position, it can be hard for the bottom to focus properly on the spanking. For some, it can interfere with pain processing techniques and distract from enjoyment. If the spanking is being given for punishment, this is a feature, not a bug. It is up to you to decide if this position meets your needs.

Furthermore, this position takes a lot of self-discipline on behalf of the bottom. The temptation to stand up or try to move away from a heavy swat can be tempting. The Top may need to reinforce their order (if you're playing with power exchange) to stay still during the scene. Some bottoms may need more positive reinforcement to stay where the Top wants them.

The skin will be stretched taut in this position, increasing the intensity of any impact. The sweet spot is also very exposed, and a miscalculation in aim could end up with genitals being hit accidentally (of course, they can also be hit intentionally, if you wish). These factors combine to make touching the toes a very intense and difficult position.

Diaper Position

The diaper position combines many of the advantages of the above positions; the bottom is laying down, the sweet spot is exposed, bondage may be employed to enhance the feeling of helplessness, and the Top is free to move as they desire. It adds an element of embarrassment or humiliation by exposing the bottom's genitals and putting them in an infantilized position.

Have the bottom lay on their back on a solid surface like a bed. Take a hold of the legs and raise them up above the bottom's head. You can use bondage to secure them into this position or you can use your shoulder and back to hold the legs in position. Your aim is to situate the bottom the same way as you would hold a baby while changing their diaper.

In this position, the sweet spot is exposed and the skin is stretched taut. This helps increase the intensity of any impact. The genitals are also exposed (or can easily be exposed by opening the legs slightly). This position can leave a bottom feeling very vulnerable and embarrassed.

Some bottoms will find this position strenuous to maintain. This is often eased by allowing them to rest their legs against your back and shoulder or by using bondage to help hold the legs in place. If too much stress is placed on the back, try a harder or softer surface, which may help ease discomfort

The Implements of Discipline

There are many different types of implements for discipline. This guide details the use and care of some of the more common ones, as well as a number of less common implements. I've tried to cover a variety of price ranges, have given options for pervertables (everyday items that can be used for kink) and a few DIY ideas.

The use of Hands

Of course, the cheapest and easiest implement is something that many of us already have. Our hands allow us to have a spur of the moment scene when we don't have any toys with us. They give us instant feedback on the intensity of our swats. They create a unique intimacy through touch. They can be used to cause pain and soothe it, over and over again.

Before getting into all the wonderful implements, let's take a moment to talk about what we can do with our hands. Spanking is often the first experience many of us have with BDSM, it's also a common first fantasy. The joy of it stays with most of us, even though we move on to discover many other ways to experience what we love, we still come back to hand spanking.

Swat with an open, flat hand against your bottom's bottom. Next, try changing the way you hold your hand as you spank. Cup your hand and see how that works. You should get a much louder noise, maybe a lighter impact. Slap with just your fingers, no palm. It turns the sensation stingy and makes a much different sound. Bring your hand back, hitting with your knuckles in a backhand slap for yet another sensation.

Swat with your whole hand but snap it back at the moment of impact. Again, you will create a stingy sensation. Press into the skin on your next swat, as if you're trying to follow through on your swing. The sensation becomes much more thuddy.

All of these sensations with the same hand. Keep going, what is the difference if you splay your fingers versus keeping them together? How many different sensations can you create using only your hands?

Use both hands. Alternate, one then the other, like playing the drums. Speed it up and slow it down. Swat with both hands at once, one on each cheek or side of the body. Notice the reaction.

Hands don't always have to be flat. You can close your hand and hit with your knuckles - not quite a punch, and do it lightly. If your bottom likes thuddy, this could be the ticket. If you want to go a bit harder, proceed slowly and only on very fleshy parts of the body like the buttocks.

Make use of your fingernails to mix things up a bit. Gentle or more intense scratching is a sensation that many people like.

Don't forget all the nice things you can do with your hands too, rubbing, massaging, stroking, tickling and more. Experiment with as much as you can to get a full understanding of the wide ranging implements you were born with.

Once you're done playing around with your hands, read on for instructions on how to use a variety implements, from the mild to the intense and easy to more complex.

Learning to Use Your Implements

There is a wide range of implements that can fall under the umbrella of "Classic Discipline", which can be used for impact play, including canes, floggers, switches and, of course, hands. With such a range of possibilities, it's good to have a general idea of what sensation each type of implement will deliver.

I always advocate for trying out your toys on your own body first - you should know for sure the relative intensity and feel of an implement will give. Hitting the inside of your arm or your calf will help you understand the intensity and type of impact (although it won't be able to help you understand how a masochists brain interprets it unless you also happen to be a masochist).

While some people believe that you should have a toy used on you - in the context of a scene or at least in earnest - before you use it on others, I don't agree. My brain interprets pain sensations differently than my bottom's brain does, which is why I'm not a bottom. Additionally, my personal disabilities prevent me from being a bottom for many BDSM activities, whether I want to engage in them or not. Should I then be prevented from Topping for those activities? Should I not be able to buy and use new toys ever again? Sounds rather silly, doesn't it?

If you find value in bottoming to a toy before you Top with it, please go ahead and do so. If that is something that does not appeal to you for any reason, then don't.

As you gain experience, you will find that certain types of implements will give similar sensations. Different materials will give different sensations. The intensity of an implement will change depending on these factors as well. With some practice and experience, you will be able to look at an implement and have a good idea of the intensity and type of sensation it will give before you even pick it up.

Implements for impact play can be divided into different categories. Short range implements (paddles, slippers, hands, etc) and long range implements (floggers, tawses, canes, etc) are one possible way to categorize them. In this system, long range implements will typically be more painful than short range implements.

Implements can also be divided by type; including stick-like implements (canes, crops or rulers), non-elastic flat implements (paddles, hairbrushes or wooden spoons), elastic flat implements (strap, tawse or slipper) and whipping implements (flogger, martinet or quirt). These categories can tell you a bit about what the implement will feel like before you use it.

Materials will also have a bearing on the feel of an implement. Suede is much softer and can deliver a lighter sensation or a thuddy one, in the case of a flogger with many falls. Rubber will always feel intense and often stingy, delivering an impact that is generally only preferred by heavy masochists.

Let's start with the implement that most of us possess - our hands. We discussed earlier the different sensations you can deliver with hands. Some of those same techniques can be applied to other implements as well. Keep in mind that snapping the implement away at the moment of impact increases the sting, so will enhance the sensation of a stingy implement. Trying to follow through on your swing will enhance the thud.

Paddles will generally deliver thuddy sensations because the impact is spread out over a larger area. You can find paddles of all shapes and sizes, made from a variety of materials. The larger the paddle, the more 'thud' it will have. Flexibility and materials also come into play. A leather paddle will generally be more thuddy than a rubber one, which would be fairly stingy. Wooden paddles will often give a quick sting followed by a lasting thuddy feeling. More flexibility will often mean a stingier paddle.

You may have seen some paddles with holes in them and wondered why. The holes help eliminate the small cushion of air that you would have in a regular paddle, making the impact more intense.

Spoons, rulers and other household 'paddle' style implements will vary in their sensations and intensity. Generally, long, thin implements will deliver a stingy sensation. Wooden spoons can range from stingy, slim spoons to thuddy, larger spoons. Lighter woods will have less intensity than heavier wood. Silicone spoons and other baking tools are fairly popular and can be found in many discount stores, making cheap and effective implements. Silicone tends to be quite intense and stingy, although some can also pack a deep thud. Wooden rulers will often be stingy since they lack the surface area and weight to deliver a good thuddy sensation. Be aware that plastic rulers can easily break, due to brittle, cheap plastic. If you want to try out a plastic ruler (and even some cheaper wooden ones), be sure that it can stand up to the unorthodox use first.

Hairbrushes fall into the same area as spoons and rulers - they can be fairly intense but cheaper ones are easily broken. Since many are made of plastic, breakage with splinters is a concern. Be sure your brush can stand up to the abuse so that you don't hurt your bottom in ways you don't intend.

In the realm of domestic discipline, the use of slippers to spank is popular. In modern times, the slippers used are often the ones with a thin rubber coating on the bottom. More historically accurate slippers would closely resemble gym shoes with a heavy rubber sole. The type of slipper will determine the sensation. Light slippers won't be very intense, just a mild sting. Heavy slippers will give more thud and intensity.

Riding crops are an iconic symbol of BDSM, and can be an inexpensive and enjoyable implement. Capable of fairly intense sensation, most crops will be used in a way that delivers a more moderate sting. The small tress will traditionally be leather, but I have crops with rubber tresses too (which are very intense and thuddy).

Canes are synonymous with discipline and can be extremely intense. Generally made of rattan, canes deliver a harsh stingy sensation and can easily break the skin if you aren't careful. There are canes being made in many materials now, but they are all long, thin and flexible. It is this flexibility that gives them both the sting and intensity that many find satisfying.

Straps and tawses (a strap with two tails) are quite intense, generally delivering a sharp sting along with an intense thud. Materials like silicone will give more sting than leather, but both will have a lingering thud. For the sake of this section, belts classify as straps and have the same qualities described here. As longer range implements, a full arm swing with a strap or tawse will be very intense and requires precise aim (a subject we will discuss in depth later in this book).

Floggers have a wide range of intensities and sensations, depending n a number of factors. The material of the flogger will do a fair bit to determine its intensity. Softer materials, like suede, will be less intense, where heavier materials like rubber will be quite intense. The weight of the falls, which can depend both on the material and the number of falls, will help determine the sensation. Heavier floggers are more thuddy, where lighter ones are often quite stingy. The cut of the falls, any finishing techniques, and their condition will also affect the sensation of the flogger. Braided falls are more stingy and generally more intense. Falls that are cut to a point will be stingier where rounded or blunted falls will lack that sting. Knotted or weighted falls will add significantly to the intensity of the flogger, although knots will create more sting, while weights create more thud. There is wide variation in floggers, which is why it's a good idea to try them out in person before purchasing one.

Martinets and cat o' nine tails are similar to floggers, but with much fewer falls. Much of what applies to floggers will apply to them as well. Both implements are generally more stingy and intense.

Quirts are a lesser known implement, looking like a cross between a whip and a flogger. They are quite intense, no matter what material they are made of. The impact is stingy with some thud, but this will vary depending on materials.

While you may be able to have a good idea of how an implement will feel before using it, it really is best to confirm your thoughts by trying it out on your own body first. As above, a few hits on the inner arm (which is more sensitive) or the inside of your calf (again, a more sensitive spot) will quickly let you know if you were right. Having an idea of the relative intensity and sensations of various implements will help you to plan a scene properly and know what you are expecting your bottom to endure.

Common Implements and Their Use

I firmly believe that in-person, hands-on instruction is the best way to learn how to learn the Topping skills that are associated with BDSM. I have shared a good base of knowledge here so that you can get started along your path and know enough that you should be able to identify appropriate instructors. Please do not let this book be your only learning experience - get out and learn from others in person, buy other books and get as much information as you can.

Canes

Canes are one of the most feared BDSM implements and with good reason. Depending on how they are used, they can break the skin and cause great pain. While this may be what we are looking for in some scenes, many people will find this distasteful and avoid canes. The truth is that with a bit of skill, canes can be used in many ways - they can be almost sensual.

Canes have been used all over the world as an implement of discipline. They are banned in many places, as societies have moved away from corporal punishment, but are still used in some parts of the world. Judicial canings are quite brutal and leave scars on those punished. Some members of the kink community will remember canings in school.

This history is part of why canes are so feared and loved in BDSM. Tops who are sadistic enjoy not only the sensations that canes cause their bottoms but the fear the implement instills.

Canes are a surface oriented implement, although some canes can be felt deeply in the body. The flexibility of canes is what makes them so powerful, the force of the swing is amplified along the length of the cane as it lands. Being aware of the hazards of this flexibility is important. When users underestimate a cane, they can easily wrap the tip around the body, causing unintended pain and damage.

Size and Materials

Canes can be made of many materials, from natural to synthetic. Some are more appropriate than others. Canes need to be strong, flexible and able to withstand the force of the blow they are delivering.

Many people look at the classic cane and think they see bamboo. Rattan and bamboo may look similar but they are very different. Bamboo dries out easily and will crack and shatter, leaving sharp shards of it in your bottom's skin. Even treated, bamboo is not safe to use (there are very few exceptions to this) due to its propensity to splinter.

Rattan is a reed that grows throughout Indonesia and the surrounding areas. It is a very traditional cane making material and is generally readily available in North America since it is used to make furniture and many other things. For canes, rattan should always have the skin on. Rattan comes in varying thicknesses and is relatively inexpensive and takes some skill to work with.

The advantage of rattan is that with proper care, it will stay supple and flexible. If it does break, it will do so cleanly, usually breaking at one of the joints, not injuring the bottom.

Fiberglas is inexpensive, light and flexible. Be careful though because the very cheap stuff can shed fibres and should be discarded when it does. Higher quality fibreglass doesn't seem to have this problem, so investing in quality is worth it.

Delrin is a black, heavy rubber like substance. Because of the weight, it can be quite thuddy, if the cane is thick enough. It is still very flexible, even with the weight. Delrin can be quite painful.

Lucite is not just for stripper heels anymore! Very rigid, so they tend to break easily and aren't a 'true' cane. Canes made from Lucite can be beautiful, they can come in any colour under the sun and have a variety of designs, such as twisted canes.

There are other materials used for canes. Pretty much anything that is long, thin and flexible could be called a cane.

Canes can come with a handle or without, it is up to the user to decide which they prefer. Handles also come in a variety of styles, from elaborate, carved wood to simple shrink foam to cushion the hand.

The type of cane will determine its dimensions. Traditional canes of different sizes have different names. Most canes will be around one meter (a little over three feet) in length, although variations do occur. The length is important so that the cane can build up enough energy through the swing to deliver the stinging blow that is intended.

Junior canes, sometimes referred to as nursery canes, are the smallest of the traditional canes. They are typically between 40 cm (16 inches) to 92 cm (36 inches) long and 6-7 mm (1/4 inch) thick. They tend to be very flexible and whippy, which makes them the most stingy of the traditional canes.

Senior canes are a little bit larger than junior canes, measuring 60 cm (24 inches) - 92 cm (36 inches) long and 8 - 10 mm (1/3 inch) thick. While they may lose a bit of flexibility due to their thickness, they are still very whip like at longer lengths. The increase in thickness only takes a slight edge off the sting of a junior cane but adds intensity.

A reformatory or punitive cane is larger still, at around 92 cm (36 inches) long and 10 - 12 mm (1/2 inch) thick. At this thickness, more of the flexibility is lost, although it is still very possible to wrap the tip of the cane. Some of the sting is exchanged for intensity. These canes are getting large enough to cause serious damage to the bottom if the Top isn't careful.

Singapore or dragon canes are the largest of the traditional canes. At 13 mm - 16 mm (1/2 - 3/5 inch) thick, they are less flexible than their smaller counterparts but by no means are they rigid. Generally, between 92 cm and 1.2 m long, they can be difficult to wield at times. These canes are large enough to cause serious harm if they aren't used properly (and even when they are used properly). Precision is incredibly important with dragon canes.

Sensation

Canes are traditionally stingy implements, although there can be some variation based on size and materials.

Thicker canes, like dragon canes, can be surprisingly thuddy, while thinner canes are more stingy. Typically, more rigid canes will deliver more thud than their flexible counterparts, which are more stingy. The length of the cane will also help determine how stingy it is. Longer canes are more whip-like, especially if they are made from a flexible material and are thin, this adds to the sting of the impact.

Canes often deliver a two-step sensation, that seems to be unique to them. The first step of this sensation is the initial sting when the cane first comes in contact with the skin. The second step comes a moment later, often as a sensation felt deeper in the body. For this reason (among others) heavy cane strikes should be spaced out and not come in rapid succession, which is often used with lighter strokes.

As discussed in the materials section, different materials will give different sensations. Rattan tends to be stingy because of its flexibility. Thick rattan canes can be thuddy, but it's usually only the thickest canes that deliver a thuddy sensation. Heavier materials, like delrin, can deliver a bit more of a thuddy sensation, but will generally still be quite stingy.

Marks

Canes leave a distinctive mark on the skin. Two raised, red parallel lines with space in between is a typical cane mark. When getting into heavier caning, these marks may simply be one long, red (or purple) welt.

Depending on intensity, marks may fade in a matter of hours and welts can take days or even weeks to heal completely. With more extreme play, where the skin is broken, scars can take years to fade and can be permanent.

Technique

Basic technique

Position your bottom where you can have access to the areas you want to cane - typically the buttocks or upper back. Make sure that you have enough space to swing your cane, especially if you are doing a heavier scene where you will be doing full arm swings. The length of canes means that you may need more space than you anticipated. Stand far enough away from the bottom that the end of the cane connects with the bottom.

Grip your cane at the base or on the handle. For canes without a handle, there may be a hanging loop to indicate the base of the cane or you may have to go with what feels right. Canes do have a specific orientation, you just have to feel it out.

It is also possible to use a cane from a seated position for Tops who have mobility or other issues that prevent or make standing difficult. You may find that you will have to adjust the position of your bottom to maintain proper form. For example, caning the buttocks is fairly easy from a seated position, even if the bottom is standing. Caning the upper back of a standing bottom would be difficult to do with proper technique. Instead, have the bottom lie down or even kneel in an appropriate spot to reach this area.

Gripping the cane comfortably in your dominant hand (although practising with your non-dominant hand is highly recommended for versatility), extend your index finger along the length of the cane. This will give you greater control over its movements. If you are planning on doing a heavy caning, you can choose whether to extend your finger or not. For the heaviest strokes, most people prefer not to extend their finger.

The cane should be an extension of your arm. By holding it the way described above, you have good control over the implement, despite its length. You should be able to strike with only the smallest movements.

Stand away from your bottom, so that when you strike, only the last 5 cm or 10 cm of the cane makes contact with the skin. You want to avoid hitting with the tip of the cane itself, instead of landing your blow so that the shaft of the cane connects with the bottom.

The cane should extend straight from your hand, in line with your arm. It should connect with your bottom to create a 90-degree angle. If your impact comes at a different angle, you could wrap the tip of the cane or even break the cane.

Warm up is especially important when it comes to canes, even if you've used other implements to warm up your bottom, it is still wise to start with light cane strokes.

The lightest strokes can be delivered by simply wiggling your extended finger. Canes flexibility will allow the cane to start wiggling up and down, giving light strikes. This technique can be effective as part of a warm up or for use on more sensitive areas of the body, such as the genitals.

To increase the intensity, move more of your hand. An average cane strike can be delivered with the wrist. A moderately intense strike will happen when you bend your elbow and straighten your arm. Full arm strikes with a cane will be very intense and require perfect aim.

You can strike a single butt cheek or both with a single stroke. Be aware of where on the cane you are connecting, keeping in mind that if you're standing too close, you will hit closer to the centre of the cane, causing wrap or breakage. If you are striking the upper back, do not try to hit both sides at once. You could land the cane on the spine, causing it damage or, more likely, breaking the skin.

Caning is dynamic, you should be moving while you strike. You will need to switch sides and possibly hands, in order to strike the opposite side of your bottom's bottom or back. Don't stand stiffly while you cane, be relaxed and don't be afraid to move around.

The backhand

It is best to practice using a cane in both hands so that you can strike the part of your bottom you want to with minimal effort. Some people will find this too difficult to master and may prefer to use a backhand swing instead. Both techniques are good to learn.

Holding the cane in the same way as above, draw it across your body to begin the strike. You will likely need to crouch down into a lunge position in order to maintain proper caning form and strike properly. Remember that your strike should make a 90-degree angle and only connect the last 5 cm - 10 cm of the cane.

Making a cane stingy(er)

If you have a thuddy cane and you want it to be a stingy strike - to keep your bottom on their toes with something they're not expecting - simply snap the cane back at the moment of impact. The movement should be a quick snap, as soon as the cane makes contact with the bottom, pull it back.

Cold caning or punishment caning

Cold caning is a punishment technique that will often raise large welts or break skin. While a few heavy masochists will enjoy this style of caning, it is generally reserved for actual punishments.

Since it is possible that you will break skin using this technique, the cane(s) used should be dedicated to the bottom and not used on anyone else. With this technique, you will be delivering hard strikes with the cane. Your aim must be perfect, a miss could seriously injure your bottom. Wrapping the tip of your cane, because of a misplaced hit (either missing your mark or hitting too low on the cane), can cause unintended injury.

Generally, a set number of strikes is decided on before beginning. You may want to have the bottom count each strike to help keep them focused on the here and now. It helps some with pain processing and lets them know how much longer they need to hold on.

Make sure you are positioned properly. You may want to secure your bottom with bondage to keep them still. Like bastinado, a misplaced strike can cause damage, so you need to be sure that your bottom isn't thrashing and moving around. Having the bottom positioned where you can bring the cane down, instead of a horizontal strike, is best. It allows you maximum control over the strike and allows you to hit hard.

Using full arm strikes, bring the cane down on the bottom's buttocks or upper back. The buttocks are a preferred site for this type of caning, but the upper back can be appropriate too if the bottom is well muscled. Pace your strikes to that they come at a predictable pace, with enough time in between for the bottom to process the sensation. You should be aiming to create a line of cane strikes, avoiding overlapping, if possible.

Where to Use

Canes can be used on many parts of the body. Beginners should stick to areas of the body that are well muscled since they are more forgiving of mistakes. The buttocks and upper back are popular places to cane, but feet (see: Bastinado), arms, legs, chest/breasts and genitals can also be caned. The face, throat/neck, top of the hands, top of the feet, stomach, and joints should be avoided.

Hard strikes to the testicles should also be avoided since the impact of a cane is very focused. You could potentially cause a rupture by hitting too hard. Light strokes are generally all you will need anyway.

Using a cane over areas of the body where the bones are close to the surface can increase the possibility of breaking the skin. Hard canings should only be done on heavily muscled areas to minimize the chance of injury.

Positions

In traditional school canings, 'boys' would be bent over a desk or a spanking horse. They can be caned with their trousers around their ankles or through their pants. 'Girls' were generally caned on their hands, and occasionally on their bottoms, with skirts up but with their bloomers on.

Religious caning would be similar to school caning, with the person being bent over a desk or other object.

Judicial caning is often done with the prisoner immobilized. They were most often bound to a frame with buttocks or back exposed to minimize movement.

Care

Canes do need special attention to ensure that they remain flexible and don't break. This care is relatively simple and will not take much time.

Canes should be stored hanging from the loop at the handle end. If your cane does not have such a loop, you can store it laying flat. Canes should never be stood on end or upright, as this will cause them to bend.

Canes need to be moisturized to keep their flexibility. It is a good idea to bring your canes into the bathroom when you have a hot shower. While they don't need to be submerged in water, the steam will help keep their moisture level where it needs to be. Once every few months should be OK unless you have a very dry home, in which case once a month might be more appropriate. Hang your canes to dry thoroughly if you store them wrapped up. A damp cane in a sealed container or wrapped in fabric can go mouldy

You may want to oil your canes occasionally - once every 6 months to a year, depending on how dry they get. Natural oils are best, but be sure to use one that won't go rancid. You can ask your cane maker what they prefer, linseed oil is the most commonly used. If you want to use a different oil, make sure that it won't turn rancid.

Discipline scenarios

Canes are ideal for a wide range of scenarios. They have been used around the world in many different contexts as a method of punishment. Keep in mind that they can be a harsh implement, so scenarios like cold caning will likely be short lived.

School roleplay is easy to do and a lot of fun. The errant student can be bent over a desk or tied to a spanking horse for punishment. They can be told to stand while their hands are caned. Add to the anticipation by having the bottom sit in a corner (dunce cap optional) while waiting for their fate to be decided. Writing lines is a tedious chore, but can be made better with an erotic twist on what's to be written.

Of course, you can always add a religious twist to a school caning scenario if you choose. Whether it's a nun punishing a student or the nun getting punished (or priest, etc), use your imagination to create a naughty, sacrilegious play scene.

Judicial caning is brutal and terrifying. We can take elements from this history to create an intense punishment or funishment scene. Read the offence and punishment out loud to the condemned to help build anticipation. Secure them to a St. Andrew's Cross, a whipping post or use your imagination to create something at home. Having your 'prisoner' lying down, well secured, will help if you're worried about squirming.

Crops

Riding crops are the quintessential BDSM implement for a Dominatrix. The classic image is a leather clad, corseted woman standing in impossibly high heels holding a crop.

Crops are a type of horse whip but work well on humans as well. Don't waste your money on buying them from a sex shop, go directly to the source and buy from a tack shop (a store that sells horse equipment). You can find a wide variety of bats (as they're called for riding), from glittery ones designed for little girls to beautiful, expensive works of art.

Size and Materials

Crops range in size from about 12 inches to 30+ inches, depending on their intended use and intended user. Crops designed for children are shorter and often decorated in whimsical ways. Some kinky folks will enjoy these, as you can get a variety of colours, textures, and shapes.

The shaft of the modern crop is made of fibreglass, although some may be other, flexible materials. The shaft is then covered in leather or fabric, by wrapping around it. The shaft thickens into the handle, made from covering the fibreglass with leather or rubber for grip. A wrist loop prevents the crop from falling when mounted.

The working end of the crop is traditionally a small piece of leather, held in place by cord. This is called a tress. Some crops that are designed specifically for BDSM will have tresses made from different materials, such as rubber. Tresses can come in a variety of sizes.

Sensation

A riding crop doesn't deliver a lot of pain, it's more of a quick sting. It does create a lovely noise, meant the get the attention of the person (or horse) on the receiving end. Of course, some crops can deliver intense sensation, bats with a rubber tress are a perfect example of this. The less intense sensation and precision mean that it is ideal for use on more sensitive body parts.

Crops are also ideal as a warm up implement, for use before moving onto more intense sensations.

The size of the tress will help determine both the stinginess and intensity of the crop, smaller tresses giving more intense, stingy sensation.

Marks

A regular riding crop should not leave lasting marks. It will create warm redness on the surface of the skin that can last a short time. Keep in mind that everyone is different, so if you have a bottom that is prone to marking, go slow until you know how they will react.

Kink-specific crops may leave bruises or welts, depending on the tress material.

Technique

Many BDSM practitioners encourage the use of the shaft of the crop, sort of like a cane. Unfortunately, this is a great way to break your crop, as they are designed for impact on the tress only. Make sure you practice with a crop so that you are only hitting with the tress, and reserve the caning for actual canes.

Crops are simple to use but do take a bit of practice to improve aim. They are a precision implement, which makes them ideal for more sensitive areas, such as nipples or genitals.

Grip the crop firmly in your dominant hand. Most strikes with a crop will be a flick of the wrist or the lower part of the arm. Full arm swings are possible, but be sure your aim is good. Starting with lighter wrist flicking blows, make sure the tress is the only part of the crop making contact. The crop is held with the top of the hand facing away from the target.

Riding crops can also be used to get the attention of the bottom or nudge their limbs into position. Use the shaft and tress to lift the bottoms head or to point and emphasize your words.

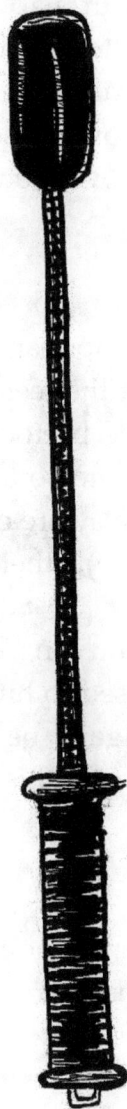

Practice

A Top should practice with the crop to ensure proper aim. Use a pillow secured at an appropriate height. The use of a fabric with nap helps you see where your blows are landing. Alternately, you can create a target to aim for on the pillow by placing a sticker or other marker. Make sure you can land blows where you are aiming more times than not before moving on to people.

Where to use

Crops can be used on most parts of the body, from the bottom of the feet and hands to the breasts or chest. Using a crop on the buttocks may not offer an intense enough sensation for some bottoms. Genitals are a popular place to use crops, just be aware of bodily fluids on the leather tress (if your crop has one), other materials may be easier to clean.

You can also use a crop to remove other items. Crops are often used to hit clothespins on the skin, in order to dislodge them. Again, be sure that you practice your aim carefully before trying this.

Positioning

Since the riding crop isn't a traditional discipline implement, there aren't specific positions to put your bottom in while using it. Any position that exposes the more sensitive parts of the body would be effective.

Care

Crops should be hung up by the wrist loop or laid flat on a surface. The tress can be cleaned with leather cleaner if leather. Non-leather parts of the crop can be cleaned using soap and water or disinfectant wipes.

Discipline Scenarios

Crops can be included in many different discipline scenarios, but are ideal for traditional English discipline. They could also be used in any sort of equestrian scenario or for Lady and Knight role plays.

Floggers

Floggers are very common in modern kink. Being able to use a flogger well is a status symbol for many Tops. The great thing about floggers is that there is a huge variety of styles, materials, and types of floggers, so there should be one to suit your needs.

Floggers do take a bit of practice to master, but it's worth the effort. Buying a flogger that is well made, balanced and suited for you will ensure that you're able to throw it with ease (and hopefully a bit of grace).

Size and Materials

Floggers can be made of a huge variety of materials, including leather, rope, rubber, silicone, horsehair, fur, suede and more. Handles are often wood, sometimes covered in the same material that the falls are made of. Each material will lend the flogger a different sensation, weight and care regimen.

The ideal size for a flogger is to have a handle that you can fit two hands on and falls that reach from your wrist to your armpit. That is a huge variation in size considering the variations in the size of people in the world. For simplicity sake, I would not recommend a flogger which is larger than the specifications above. Smaller floggers may be a bit more difficult for some people to learn, but they are more easily controlled than ones that run larger.

Floggers also need to be balanced. The handle may need to be weighted to counter the weight of the falls. The balance point should be an inch or two (depending on the size) behind where the falls meet the handle. This will make the flogger easier to handle and take less energy to swing.

Falls should be uniformly cut and of equal length. They can be finished with different cuts, such as rounded, ribbon, angled or blunt. Beads, weights or knots may be added to the ends to alter the sensation.

In addition to the traditional style floggers, where the falls meet a handle in a smooth transition, there are alternative styles you may want to try out. Swivel handled floggers have a solid handle which attaches to a swivel which then attaches to the falls. Use of these floggers is slightly different, but they can be used for all of the techniques described below. Poi style handles are simply two finger loops. The falls may be attached to these loops by a short rope, chain or a swivel. The use of these is similar to traditional floggers but may appeal to those who already have a solid knowledge in the use of poi.

Sensation

With the wide variety of materials, as well as variations in style and size, it would take pages to describe the sensations possible through flogging.

There are a few general rules that can be observed in regards to the sensation of a flogger.

- A greater number of falls means a more thuddy sensation. Fewer falls means a more stingy sensation.
- Wider falls offer a more thuddy sensation, while thinner ones are more stingy.
- Falls finished with a blunt or rounded cut will give a more thuddy feeling. Angled or ribbon cut falls will be more stingy.
- Weighted falls will be more thuddy and increase the intensity.
- Beaded falls will be more stingy and increase the intensity. Heavier beads will act like weights.
- Knotted falls will add to the sting. Some knots are designed to increase the 'damage' that a flogger does and can cause bruising or even break the skin.
- Braided falls will be more stingy.
- The stiffer material will add to sting, softer material will give more thud.

Leather floggers are by far the most common. Depending on the factors above, they can range from stingy to thuddy, less intense to very intense and everything in between. A good leather flogger is a staple of many toy bags (although there are a lot of options for people who don't use animal products too).

Suede floggers, soft leather floggers (like deer or moose hide) are generally quite thuddy. They are often designed with many falls, sometimes called a 'mop', to increase the thuddy quality. They can range from medium to heavy intensity.

Fur floggers are great for warm up. They are all thud, often quite soft and have less intensity. They are great for sensation oriented scenes as well as a starter flogger for funishment scenes.

Rubber and silicone floggers are notorious for being quite intense. They can range from stingy to thuddy. These are ideal for masochists and other heavy pain players.

Rope floggers are generally stingy. The thickness of the rope can add or take away from this sensation. Some warm up floggers are made from nylon rope that has been untwisted and perform similarly to fur floggers, including having a thuddy feel.

Marks

Most floggers won't leave marks beyond a bit of redness that should fade over 30 minutes to two hours (depending on skin type). It generally takes a lot of work to leave bruises or other marks with a flogger if used correctly.

Wrapping a flogger can cause welts that can take hours to days to heal. Wrapping should be avoided and is regarded as a mistake in technique. A few people have mastered the art of controlling the wrap and can wrap a flogger on purpose to hit a mark on the other side of the body. This takes a high level of skill and practice and should not be attempted by anyone but experts in the field due to the probability of error and injury.

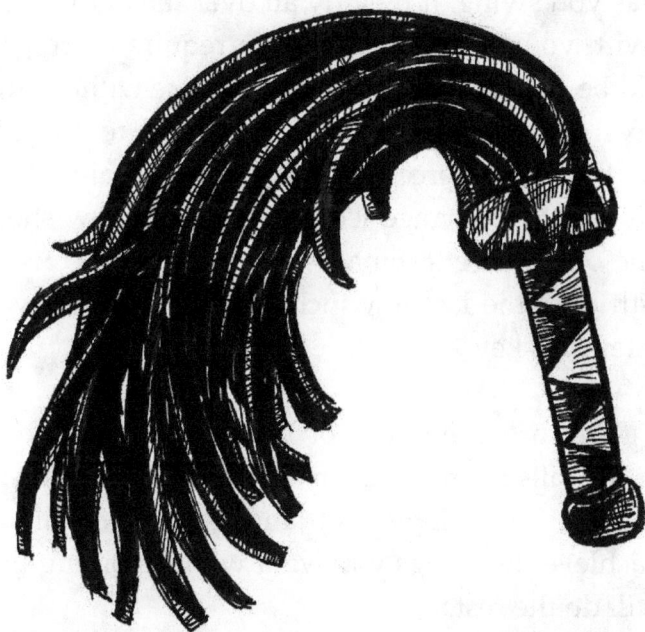

Heavy rubber floggers, weighted falls, and knotted falls can leave bruises when used in heavy play. Very thin and stiff falls on a flogger can cause welts or in extreme cases cut the skin. This is more likely when used on skin where the bones are closer to the surface.

Technique

There are a wide variety of flogging techniques. We will go over the basics here, which will give you skills to use to create a full flogging scene. From circles for warm up, figure 8's for mid-range play and overhand strikes for more intense play, these three techniques can be combined to achieve a full range of sensation.

There are few very important things to remember when using a flogger. The falls should stay together in a relatively tight grouping as you swing, if they fly all over the place, there is a problem with your technique and you require more practice. You should be able to flog as long as you like without the falls splaying everywhere. You should also be able to hit the same spot, with the same force, over and over again. Basically, unless you decide to change techniques, each blow should be just like the one before it. Finally, you should be consistently hitting with only the last few inches of the falls. As you can see, consistency is key.

Similarly, there are a number of things you want to avoid. Wrapping the falls is one of them, as is hitting wildly and not knowing where your blows will land. Proper technique will help you achieve the things you want while avoiding the bad. Practice will do the rest.

When using a flogger, it is important to avoid wrapping the falls around the body, which is why we only hit with the last few inches of the falls. Wrapping happens when we hit with the middle of the falls and the ends wrap around a leg, arm or the torso. This causes the ends to move much quicker than intended, and they land with much more force than you will want. This can cause an unintended degree of pain for the bottom - one that they find too much or beyond their limits. It can also break skin and leave nasty welts or other marks. Depending on where you wrapped, these marks can be an issue for day to day life. Imagine a bottom having to explain welts or bruises on their face due to an 'accident'.

When flogging, you should be standing comfortably, feet shoulder width apart. If you want to change where you hit, you should move your whole body, move your feet and position yourself appropriately. Do not just lean in or over. If you can not move your body to the right spot, move your bottom.

Flogging from a seated position is possible for Tops with mobility (or other) issues that prevent them from standing. Many of the techniques here can be adjusted to accommodate seated flogging with only minor adjustments.

There are a few ways to grip a flogger. Experiment with them and find what is comfortable for you. You may find that for one technique, one grip style is more comfortable while a different grip is better for a different technique.

Grip the flogger firmly but comfortably in your dominant hand, in the middle of the handle. You shouldn't have a death grip on the flogger but you don't want it to fly out of your hand on the first swing either! Keep your wrist relaxed and loose, so that the flogger points downwards when your arm is by your side.

Another way to hold your flogger that works well with the circle and figure 8 techniques is to place the end of the handle between your middle and ring finger. You should have two fingers on either side of the handle. Close your hand around the end knot if there is one. This really only works with floggers that have a larger knot (known as a Turk's head knot) or other knobs on the end. Again, make sure your wrist is relaxed and loose.

Sometimes you may find that gripping the back end of the handle (away from the falls) is most comfortable. I have a few floggers where this is the case, they all tend to be shorter, lighter floggers.

Don't put your hand through the belt/hanging loop on the end of the flogger. This is only for hanging the flogger, not a wrist strap to stop the flogger from flying out of your hand. Using the strap in this way will interfere with the proper motion of the flogger.

Flogging is a fairly energy-intensive activity for the Top. With proper technique and well made, balanced floggers, you can minimize the energy expended and maximize the sensation for the bottom. This means that you can spend a much longer time flogging if you so choose. Poor technique and improperly balanced floggers often result in a Top who gets tired quickly from inefficient action.

Circles

Circles are a great warm up technique. They also help the Top become comfortable letting their wrist do a lot of the work of flogging. This is a good way to master keeping the falls together.

The motion here is similar to using a jump rope. In fact, jumping rope is a great way to practice flogging when you can't be seen using a flogger - and you get some cardio exercise too.

Begin by bringing your arm up to your side. Your elbow should be about waist height. Resist the temptation to lock your elbow in close to your body or rest it on your hip. Keep your arm relaxed and a comfortable distance from your body.

Start to swing the flogger in a circle, with most of the motion in your wrist. You can do both forward circles and backward ones, so begin with whichever feels most comfortable. This is meant to be a continuous motion, so don't just go around once and stop.

Keep making circles and see how long you can go for. You will begin to feel a strain on the muscles in your forearm. This is normal, it will take some time to build up your stamina and muscle memory. You may even have a bit of soreness the next day, in the same way that you would if you went to the gym.

Experiment with the speed too. There is a lower threshold for speed, if you fall below this point, the falls won't stay together. If you're doing them right, your flogger should be spinning in a circle beside you, with all of the falls together neatly.

Practising both forward and backward circles are important since each one has useful applications when it comes to play. Forward circles hit the bottom in a downward motion, so are ideal for flogging the shoulders and chest. Of course, they can be used on other parts of the body as well but work best for those areas. Backward circles hit the bottom in an upward motion, which makes them ideal for the buttocks. The upward motion catches the roundness of the buttocks and hits the sweet spot.

Circles are great for warm ups because they are a fairly light and rhythmic technique. This allows the bottom to become accustomed to the sensation. The predictability of knowing when the next blow will land can help nervous bottoms relax - they know what to expect next. Many people find that a consistent rhythm is helpful or even needed to enter into subspace.

The intensity can be altered slightly by slowing down or speeding up your circles. You can also add emphasis to the swing with your wrist when it comes in contact with your partner but be careful not to change how much of the flogger you're hitting with.

Figure 8's

Figure 8's have a lot of the same benefits of circles. They result in a predictable rhythm of blows and don't take a lot of energy on the part of the Top. This technique combines a forehand and backhand swing to create a continuous, fluid motion. Figure 8's can be used to hit both sides of the body - one with the forehand swing and the other with the backhand. They can also be tightened up to hit repeatedly in the same spot.

This technique requires the wrist to be loose since this is where a large part of the motion will come from. Using your shoulder and elbow, draw the flogger across the front of your body in a downward diagonal motion. Use your wrist to change direction and return the flogger to the starting point in an upward diagonal motion. Effectively, you are drawing a sideways 8 or infinity sign in the air in front of you.

Keeping your wrist loose and your motion fluid is important to mastering this technique. Once again, this is meant to be a continuous motion, so don't stop with just one figure 8.

Ideally, the flogger should be coming into contact with the bottom during the diagonal part of the swing. For a right handed Top, hitting the right side on the downward diagonal swing and the left side on the upward diagonal swing.

By lengthening the swing, you can hit both sides of the body, such as both cheeks of the buttocks or both shoulder blades. By tightening up your swing, you can hit the same spot or the same side of the body with your swing.

Practice this technique in each hand to prepare yourself to learn Florentine style flogging, which uses two matching floggers at once. This advanced technique is hard to describe through text and won't be included because of that. It's one of those things better learned via in-person instruction or even through video.

Towel Snap

This technique is almost exactly like the towel snap that many of us used as kids/young adults.

Bring the flogger across your body, gathering the falls in your other hand. Quickly extend your arm towards the bottom using your elbow. At the point where the ends of the falls come in contact with your bottom, snap your arm back towards your body. This will cause the falls to move quickly and just 'kiss' the skin.

This technique is going to deliver a much more stingy sensation, even if you are using an otherwise thuddy flogger. It's a great way to get your bottom's attention or mix things up without switching toys.

Overhand or Heavy Swings

There are times when you want to get your bottom's attention or impart some heavy sensation. Overhand swings are ideal for this.

Holding the flogger firmly in your hand, bring it up and over your shoulder on the same side. You can use your other hand to gently gather the falls if you wish. Bring the flogger down in a slightly diagonal direction. You can let gravity do the work for a lighter blow or add some muscle for a more impactful one. The swing should end with the flogger on the opposite side of your body with your hand pointing downwards. Contact should be made at the top of the downward motion.

Make sure that the falls stay together for the duration of the swing. You will also need to be sure that you are positioned far enough away from your bottom that you hit with only the last few inches of the falls, to avoid wrapping. You should not try this technique until you are confident in your ability to aim consistently - hitting the back of the bottom's head or neck shows you need much more practice on an inanimate object.

Backhand Heavy Swing

The backhand heavy swing is very similar to the overhand swing, just reversed. It delivers the same intense sensation. It's great for hitting the opposite side of the body, in combination with the overhand swing.

Bring the flogger across your body and over the opposite shoulder, so the side that isn't holding the flogger. You can use your other hand to gently gather the falls if you wish. Swing the flogger down in a diagonal direction, either letting gravity do most of the work or adding in some muscle for a more intense strike. Again, contact should be made at the top of the swing. At the end of the swing, your arm should be straight alongside your body.

If the falls don't stay together, you may need to speed up your swing or practice more - possibly both. If you hit too far down on the falls, you can wrap the falls over the shoulder or even around the neck. This can be avoided with practice and making sure to contact only with the last few inches of the falls (I know I've been repetitive, but it's important!).

Practice

Like many of the other implements, it is important to practice on a pillow or other inanimate object until your aim is reliable. Practice each new technique for as long as it takes to be able to consistently hit your mark without mistakes.

I suggest learning these techniques in the order that they are listed in this book. Circles, followed by figure 8's to start. You can then add in your towel snaps and finally your overhand and backhand swings for intensity. You don't need to know all of the techniques to start working flogging into your scenes. If you've practised circles enough to feel comfortable trying it on a real bottom, you can use them as a warm-up, then switch to other implements for other parts of the scene.

You can use a pillow covered in fabric that has a nap. This refers to material that leaves an impression when you run your hand over it in one direction and erases the impression if you rub it the other way. This way you can see where you've hit and can adjust your aim until it's perfect. You can also use some rope or ribbon to divide the pillow into quarters so that you can focus on a smaller area to hone your skill.

Be sure to adjust the height of the pillow. Secure it to the back of a chesterfield to simulate a bent over bottom. Use the seat of a chair to simulate a bottom laying down or the back of the chair to mimic the height of a bottom's buttocks while standing. To get some practice on shoulder height targets tie the pillow to a coat rack, bookcase or anything else that will get it to the correct height.

The first thing you should practice is the general motion of the swing you are trying to learn. Don't worry about aim or where the falls are going at first, just make sure you have the proper form. Standing, relaxed with your feet shoulder width apart. Begin your swing without a target. Just get the motions committed to memory while flogging the air.

If you need to be seated, find a chair to sit on that doesn't have arms for the floggers falls to get caught on - a stool is ideal if you are comfortable on one. If you use a wheelchair, remove any parts, if possible, that the flogger could catch. Once you have better control over the flogger, this may not be necessary.

When you feel comfortable with the motions, set up your pillow or other targets. Begin by placing your body in the correct position, but a little too far away. This next step is easier to do when standing, rather than sitting, so do what works best for you. Begin your swing, taking note of how much space there is between the end of the falls and your target. While still swinging the flogger, take a step forward. Try to judge how much distance you need to close before the ends of your flogger hit the target.

If the falls begin to wrap around the target or get tangled in it, you've moved too far. If you are barely making contact, you haven't gone far enough (although it can be fun to tease a bottom with the lightest touch of the flogger or even the wind it creates). This will help you learn the length of your flogger. When you move on to people, you should still start in this way to avoid accidents.

When it's time to move on to practice on your bottom, try placing a scarf, towel or even another toy over the parts you don't want to hit. If your bottom is standing or kneeling for a shoulder/upper back flogging, place a towel around the back of their neck. This will help protect them from an errant swing and let you know if you've missed. The sound of a flogger hitting skin vs a towel is quite different. If your bottom is bent over to expose their buttocks, place the towel over their tailbone and hips. Again, you will quickly hear the difference if you miss.

When you're first starting out, you should stick to a single flogger. Get to know how it feels, how long it is, etc. Don't confuse yourself by trying to learn with five different floggers of varying weights and sizes. It's great to use different floggers in a single scene, but don't make learning harder than it has to be.

Each time you buy a new flogger, I suggest you break out the pillow and practice your aim. Each flogger is different so it makes sense to try it out on something you don't have to apologize to when you miss. Nothing makes bottom lose confidence quicker than being hit in the back of the head with a flogger.

Where to use

Floggers feel best over large areas of the body where there is muscle. This is why the upper back/shoulders and buttocks are ideal. There is enough space for the falls to land without wrapping. There aren't any bones close to the surface to give unpleasant sensations.

When flogging the upper back, you want to be careful of wrapping. It's easy to do in this area and you could hit your bottom in the face. Aim for the centre of each shoulder blade, avoiding the spine. Don't go too far down the back, below the ribs is less protected and won't feel very good to most bottoms.

The buttocks are ideal for flogging, but wrapping can be an issue here too. Wrapping the falls around the side of the hips is common and generally unpleasant. Feel free to flog the upper thighs as well, again being careful not to wrap around the sides of the legs. Stop a few inches above the knee, since flogging joints is a no-no.

You can also flog the chest and/or breasts. It is best to use lighter floggers that tend to the stingy side of sensation, rather than thuddy ones. Obviously, you will want your bottom to hold their head back so that you don't accidentally hit them in the face. It is generally a good idea to go a bit easier on the chest, at least until you know how your bottom will respond.

You can flog both the arms and legs if you want to. A smaller flogger will make this a lot easier since the smaller surface area means wrapping can be an issue. Remember to go a bit easier on the underside of arms or the inside of the legs. These areas are more protected day to day and won't be as 'tough' as other parts of the body.

You can also flog genitals if you like. For this, I prefer a much smaller flogger, with falls about 10 cm (just under 4 inches) in length. I also prefer to use a flogger made from easily cleanable materials. I have a silicone flogger, bought at a sex shop, for this purpose. It's simple to clean after use and will stand up to hospital grade disinfectants. Another option would be to tie a rope flogger and wash the rope when you're done.

Positions

As mentioned earlier in this section, there are a variety of positions that work well for flogging. Standing up works well for most areas of the body. It is my preferred position for flogging the upper back. The bottom can be secured to a St. Andrew's Cross, a whipping post, door frame, spreader bar and suspension point - just about anything you can think of. They can also stand without being secured, perhaps ordered to stay still with hands behind their head.

Bent over positions work nicely for flogging the buttocks, but also give access to the upper back. A spanking bench or pony is ideal for this but bent over the back of the chesterfield works wonders as well.

If you have a shorter flogger and are well practised with its use, the diaper position can work too. The flogging will be more concentrated on the upper thighs, so remember to use lighter strokes.

Lying down also gives access to the body, both front, and back. It also doesn't require any dungeon equipment at all.

Have the bottom lie on the bed, chesterfield or a massage table for access to whatever area you want to flog.

Bondage is optional in any of these positions. It is something to consider if your bottom squirms a lot. You don't want them moving in anticipation of a heavy hit, which could cause you to miss your target.

Care

Floggers should be stored hanging - that's what the loop on the end is for. This helps keep all of the falls together and stops them from getting tangled and creased. It also allows them to dry if they have gotten wet or after cleaning. If they dry laying flat, your falls could get kinked at a strange angle or wetness could more easily wick up into the handle and damage the glue holding things together.

If you are unable to hang your floggers or wish to transport them to a party or play space, use a towel. Lay the towel flat and place the flogger on top. Roll the towel up with the flogger inside. Secure the towel with elastics, string or ribbon to keep it together. You can then fold the wrapped flogger in half for easier storage. This will prevent the falls from tangling and will keep them from getting bent out of shape.

Cleaning will depend on the material of the flogger.

Rubber, silicone and other synthetic materials can be wiped down with a cleaning wipe. This will remove surface dirt, sweat and oils from the skin. If your flogger has been exposed to blood or sexual fluids, you may want to spray it down with hospital grade disinfectant. Silicone may be put in the dishwasher, but be careful if your flogger contains other materials.

Rope floggers can be cleaned with some soap and water to remove dirt, sweat, and oils. If it's really soiled, or if it has come into contact with sexual fluids, you could try washing it in a washing machine with bleach. Make sure you put it in a netted lingerie bag first. You may have to re-tie the flogger after this, so I only suggest doing this with rope floggers you've tied yourself.

Leather and suede are a bit trickier. They can be hung in sunlight to dry them out. This may also kill some bacteria that have found their way onto the leather. If you want to clean your flogger, use saddle soap or leather cleaner, following the directions on the package. Make sure you hang your flogger to dry when you're done.

Scenarios

Flogging has a number of discipline scenes that it can work for.

Floggers are used in a judicial setting. Have the prisoner restrained in a standing position, either bound to a frame or whipping post. You can also order them to their knees, hands behind their head, for the punishment. Judicial flogging is going to be concentrated on the upper back. You may wish to use a Cat O'Nine Tails, a type of flogger (see it's entry under Less Common Implements) for these scenes.

School floggings will be targeted at the buttocks. Have the misbehaving student bent over teacher's desk, holding onto the seat of a chair or secured to a spanking bench or pony. Lift up skirts or pull down pants, leaving the underwear around the ankles to add to the humiliation

Religious themed floggings can combine the above two scenarios.

Kitchen Implements

Kitchen implements make wonderful pervertables and are easy to find. Many can be bought at dollar or discount stores, so they're also quite cheap. All it takes is a bit of imagination!

Size and Materials

There is a huge range of materials available for kitchen implements.

Silicone is currently very popular in kitchen tools. It also makes for toys that have a big, thuddy impact. Cooking spoons, spatulas, and other similar tools will work as paddles.

Wooden spoons are also a popular choice, bringing back memories of childhood punishment for many people. Be careful with some of the cheaper spoons, as they can break and splinter. Bamboo cooking implements are a bit more sturdy, lightweight and cheap to buy. They are, in my opinion, a better choice.

Chopsticks can be fun to play with too. Metal chopsticks can be warmed or cooled by placing in a bowl of water and used against the skin for temperature play. The addition of two elastics on either end of a pair of chopsticks turns them into a simple set of clamps that can be used on nipples or tongues. A single chopstick can be used to poke and prod the flesh of your bottom.

With a good imagination, wandering through the kitchen section of any store should provide a plethora of kinky ideas.

Sensation

Obviously, the sensation of an implement is going to vary based on what it is, what it's made of and how it's used. In general, silicone tends to be quite thuddy and intense. Wood and bamboo is lighter and has less thud than silicone, but can be quite intense with heavy application. If using chopsticks and elastics for clamps, the tightness of the elastics will determine the intensity of the clamp.

Marks

Kitchen tools used for impact can leave bruises if you hit hard enough. Most will just leave red marks, so go a bit lighter if you are worried about leaving a more lasting impression.

Technique

For specific techniques, it's best to look at the sections that closest resemble the way you plan on using the implement. For example, if you are using a spoon as an impact toy, check the section on paddles for specific techniques.

Positioning

You can use kitchen tools when the bottom is in any position. Since they are commonly associated with childhood punishments, that style of positioning is ideal. Over the knee spanking with a wooden spoon will delight many who are into the idea of 'domestic discipline'. Diaper position adds an element of embarrassment to the punishment/funishment being doled out.

Care of Kitchen Tools

Soap and water are the best way to clean these implements or you can use antibacterial wipes. Most can even go in the dishwasher if you have one.

It is wise to keep separate tools, one set for actually cooking and one set for play - especially if you're using porous materials like wood or bamboo.

Scenarios

Kitchen tools are best for domestic style scenes. Think 1950's inspired, which can work no matter what the genders of the players, if you're willing to be inventive. Evil babysitter, cousin or other age-play scenarios can work as well.

Paddle

Paddles are a common and popular implement in BDSM. Paddles are simple to use and come in a wide variety of shapes and sizes, delivering a wide variety of sensations. Price points range from low to high, meaning that paddles are not only great for those on a budget, but also for the high-end player as well.

Size and Materials

Paddles have a huge range of sizes and materials. Most paddles are designed to be a one handed implement, although some two handed paddles exist. While these are generally considered to be a joke implement, two-handed paddles are occasionally used in BDSM play.

Paddles consist of a handle and a blade. The handle is short, designed to be gripped comfortably in one hand. It is usually 15-20 cm long. The blade is usually two or three times the length of the handle, so 30 - 60 cm long. Of course, there are paddles which are much longer. The width of the blade will depend on the intent of the paddle. Sometimes the blade will be the same width as the handle (often with little or nothing to separate the two). Some paddles will have a wide blade, between 1/3 and 1/2 of its length.

Some paddles will have holes drilled into them. These holes have two purposes; to cut down on 'wind resistance' and to eliminate the cushion of air that forms between the paddle and the site of impact. This has the effect of intensifying the sensation that the paddle delivers. A paddle with holes is going to hurt more than a paddle without.

Wood is the most common material for paddles, the type of wood making slight changes to the sensation of the paddle. The wood can then be painted or stained and sealed. Many wooden paddles are made of higher quality wood and showcase the grain with a glossy finish. If looking at a wooden paddle, be sure that it is built properly - the right type of wood, a good thickness, etc so that it won't break under 'heavy' use.

Other materials that are common for paddles include leather, rubber, silicone, metal, acrylic, vinyl, and plastic.

Leather paddles will often be reinforced with a flexible metal shank so that they maintain their shape and integrity in use. Some will have more prominent stitching which can be felt by the bottom. A well made and cared for leather paddle can last for years. The sensation it delivers may change slightly over time as it is broken in.

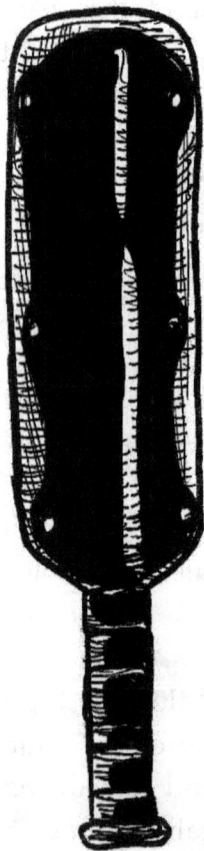

Rubber paddles come in a variety of shapes and sizes, including paddles made from the tread of a boot. They are often textured to add to the sensation. Keep in mind that the texturing of the rubber will change the sensation it delivers, often concentrating the impact on a smaller area and increasing the intensity. Considering that rubber already delivers a fairly intense sensation, you may want to ease up when using a rubber paddle or ensure that your bottom enjoys intense play.

Silicone paddles are similar to rubber. The materials are quite similar in the sensations they provide and the styles that they come in. Silicone is a great

BDSM material because it's so easy to clean, either in the dishwasher or in hot water with a bit of soap.

Metal paddles are most often seen in steel and aluminum. Some have designs in the metal, others have artwork etched onto them. Metal paddles often inspire fear in bottoms, both because they look impressive and because they deliver quite an impact.

Vinyl paddles are often sold through sex stores and online. They are often of poor or questionable quality, although some are well made. Vinyl paddles are often sold with words cut out so that it leaves a red mark in the shape of 'slut' or 'naughty' on the bottom. Vinyl paddles will generally not survive repeated use or hard use, so may be better suited for the occasional player. It is best to buy vinyl paddles in person so you can evaluate the quality of the item for yourself.

Plastic paddles, like vinyl, come in a range of quality, with most being on the low end. Plastic is generally a rigid material, which means it can easily break during heavy use. You may be able to find some higher quality plastic paddles, although it is best to shop in person for the same reason as above.

Acrylic is becoming more popular as a paddle material. While it can be brittle, depending on size and quality, it is liked for the huge variety of colours and designs that are possible. Very much like plastic and vinyl implements, buying in person can help avoid the lower quality items.

Sensation

Paddles are meant to deliver a spread out, thuddy sensation. The material of the paddle will have a large effect on the sensation, as will the size of the paddle.

In general terms, a paddle that is large, heavy and made from rigid materials will deliver a thuddy sensation. A paddle that has a small impact surface is light and made from flexible materials will be stingy. An implement that is a combination of the two lists will often lean more to the thuddy or stingy side. Some very special implements will offer a sting followed by a deep thud, giving the best (or worst) of both worlds.

Marks

Paddles will redden the skin quite quickly. Since the impact is generally spread out, they won't leave lasting marks unless used with a high level of intensity. Hitting hard will sometimes result in large, spread out bruises.

Paddles with a cutout pattern will sometimes leave the impression of the cutout on the skin. Generally, this only happens after a hard impact. Paddles with studs or texture can leave more concentrated bruising.

Technique

Always keep in mind that using an implement will create a more intense sensation than using your hand alone. Be sure to hold back and not swing too hard in the beginning. A gradual increase in intensity is just as important with paddles as it is with other implements.

Make sure the flat, wide part of the paddle comes in contact with the bottom. You want to focus on hitting with the middle of the paddle, not near the edges. On longer paddles, hitting too close to the handle can cause stress that can lead to breaks.

It is also important to move around the point of impact, rather than concentrating it in one area only. This will increase your bottom's ability to process the sensation and prolong your play time.

You can vary the sensation of a paddle slightly by changing your swing. Pulling back immediately after impact, in a sort of snapping motion, will add a sting to it. Even with a thuddy paddle, this technique will add variety. Following through or pressing against the bottom when striking can increase the thuddy-ness of the impact.

Practice

Practice your aim with a pillow secured at the appropriate height. You likely won't need to practice for very long, since paddles are basically an extension of the arm. They are easy to control and the rigidity means they move in a predictable manner. Just remember to start slowly and lightly, as harder swings can cause a loss of control.

Where to Use

Paddling is ideal for the buttocks. Thuddy impacts work best on areas of the body that have a good deal of muscle and fat to absorb the impact. The buttocks and upper thighs fit this description perfectly. They also provide a larger area of impact for larger paddles.

With that said, paddles can also be used on the upper back, tops of the thigh and even the bottoms of the feet. You will need to lighten the impact in these areas to avoid damage.

It is best to avoid using paddles on breast tissue since the impact can penetrate deep into the tissue (the thuddy sensation) and cause calcifications. Avoid using paddles in areas of the body where the bones are closer to the surface.

Positioning

Traditional paddling positions are ones where the bottom is bent over. They could be bent over a couch, sprawled over the knee of the Top, or secured to a spanking bench. By being bent over, the buttocks is more exposed as the target. The further the bottom is bent over, the more intense the sensation of the paddle will be felt, an important thing to keep in mind.

For Tops and bottoms who enjoy humiliation or age play, the diaper position is also an effective and traditional pose for paddling. This position will expose more of the upper thighs as well as the sweet spot.

Paddle Care

Much of paddle care is going to depend on the material of the paddle.

For leather paddles, cleaning with saddle soap when needed is appropriate. This will both clean and condition the leather.

For most other types of paddle, wash with a damp cloth and soap. Don't fully submerge wooden paddles in water, but plastic, rubber, silicone, acrylic and vinyl paddles can be placed in soapy water for short periods of time. Metal paddles can be cleaned in the same way, but be aware that some can rust on contact with water.

For non-porous materials, you can sanitize with hospital grade cleaning sprays such as cavicide. Silicone paddles can be placed in a dishwasher to clean.

Paddles don't require much care other than cleaning. They can be stored hanging up or packed away in bins once dry.

Paddle Scenarios

Paddles are ideal for scenarios involving school discipline. Bend the offending 'student' over the 'teacher's' desk, secure them to a spanking pony or bench or deliver the paddling while they try to stand still.

Age play scenes also lend themselves well to paddling. The paddle can be the sole form of funishment or can be one tool in a parade of parental style discipline.

Strap

There is a wide variety of straps, ranging from classic materials such as leather to modern materials like silicone. They are a single, flexible strip of material which sometimes has a handle. They are a generally intense implement that is used in many forms of classic discipline.

Straps of all descriptions were traditionally used in both school discipline and judicial corporal punishment. Straps were used in both schools and prisons in countries like Canada well into the modern era.

This category also includes items such as razor strops, belts. slappers and tawses.

Size and Materials

Straps are made from many different materials, although leather is most common. Canadian school straps are made from rubberized canvas, while some BDSM straps are made from materials like silicone.

A tawse is a strap made of leather which has two or more tongues. Slappers have two layers of leather, which slap against each other to make a loud noise. Slappers may be split into multiple tongues as well. Razor strops are the traditional leather strap used to sharpen straight razors.

Straps need to be long enough to be flexible when you swing them, but short enough not to 'bite back'. Most are in the 20 - 75 cm range, with sizes in the middle being most common. The width of a strap will also vary, from 8 to 20 cm, although some may be larger.

Sensation

Straps of all sorts are meant to deliver a stinging blow that will be remembered. Heavier straps will combine this sting with a bit of thud. Slappers are less intense than a strap of similar size.

Like any implement, the intensity can be altered by the person wielding it. Lighter strokes will give a less intense, yet still stingy blow. Harder strokes will deliver a very intense sensation, mixing sting and thud and often leaving the bottom off balance.

Some straps designed with holes in the leather, for more severe punishment. The holes prevent any cushion of air from forming between the strap and the skin. These straps are designed to leave large welts and marks.

Marks

Straps will generally cause raised red welts, especially if they have holes in them (described above). With lighter blows, these marks should fade within a few hours. Harder blows can leave welts and bruising that takes days or weeks to fade.

Be aware that heavy strokes with a strap can break the skin, as can misplaced or poorly landed blows.

Technique

There are a few main techniques used with straps. Which one you use will depend on the type of strap you have and the material it's made of. You should be aiming to strike with the last 10 to 15 cm of the strap.

Straps that are used on the buttocks or back are used by drawing the strap down onto the bottom or diagonally across the body. There should be 'follow through' with the stroke.

For bottoms that are in a laying down position, hold the strap above and slightly behind the head and forcefully bring it down until it connects. Continue the stroke until the strap arm is straight. Lessening the range of motion of the arm will give less intensity to the impact, as will moving the strap slower. For very intense strokes, bringing the strap down quickly and forcefully will deliver a blow that won't soon be forgotten.

If you have the bottom in a bent over or standing position, with the intention to strike the back or buttocks, a diagonal motion is generally easier and more accurate. Hold the strap over the shoulder of the hand holding the strap and draw it diagonally across the body, connecting with the bottom about halfway through. This technique can also be used in a backhanded manner, by starting with the strap over the opposite shoulder. Again, intensity can be regulated by shortening the stroke length and the force behind the blow. The motion is very similar to the flogging techniques of the same name.

Some straps are better used with a chopping motion. The techniques are the same as above, except that as the blow lands, the arm should be pulled back to the starting point. This helps prevent scuffing softer leathers and changes the nature of the impact, generally making it sting more.

For lighter, more continuous strokes with a strap, you can draw it back and forth, horizontally across the bottom's body. You can also use the figure eight technique, similar to what is described in the section on flogging.

Tawses were traditionally used on the hands. Many other types of strap may be used in this way as well. Have the bottom present one hand, supported by the other hand held underneath. This helps prevent the bottom from flinching and moving their hand, as well as supporting it against the blow. These strikes should not involve the full range of motion used in the earlier techniques. Bringing the strap straight down, using only the wrist and elbow is appropriate for hand strapping. Again, a shorter range of motion and less force or speed will lessen the intensity.

Practice

It is important to practice using a strap on a pillow or other inanimate object before using it on a person. Misplaced blows can cause welts, bruising, cuts and other damage. Be sure you know exactly where a strike will land before using a strap.

Be aware that the flexibility of the strap means it is prone to wrapping. Do not strike in such a manner that the end of the strap wraps around the body, as this can be very painful and cause unintended skin damage.

Finally, make sure that the strap is not landing on its edge. This can break the skin due to the concentrated impact. It is also painful and an unpleasant sensation for most bottoms.

Where to Use

Use of the strap is most common on the fleshy, well-muscled parts of the body, such as the upper back and buttocks. Straps can be used with less intensity on the chest/breasts. Some straps are traditionally used on the hands and may also be used lightly on the soles of the feet.

Positioning

Strapping the hands may be done with the bottom standing or seated, whichever the Top prefers.

When strapping other parts of the body, it is wise to brace the bottom in some way. They can lie on a bed or other surface, which will provide support and a small degree of comfort. When used for school or judicial discipline, the bottom would be bound to a whipping post with arms overhead or a punishment (spanking) horse. Bending the bottom over a table or desk will also give the support you're looking for without specialized BDSM equipment.

Care

Straps should be cleaned and moisturized regularly to keep them in top form. Depending on how often you use the strap and your local conditions (humidity, etc), this can be done once a month or once every few months.

Saddle soap is a widely accepted leather cleaner and is appropriate to use on leather straps. A glycerine soap may also be used since it is more gentle on both the skin of the person cleaning the strap and the leather itself.

Use a leather conditioner to replace the oils removed by the soap. Apply this to the leather in small, circular motions with a cloth. You may wish to finish the process with a few drops of mineral oil, to give the leather a nice shine.

Rubber coated straps, as well as silicone straps, can be washed with soap and water. Silicone straps may also be placed in the dishwasher.

Discipline Scenarios

As mentioned earlier, straps were used for both school and judicial discipline. Strapping a 'student's' hands is a typical Scottish school punishment. A fixed number of strokes - up to 36 - divided between the hands was often used to discipline students. Straps were also used on both the clothed and bare buttocks in some schools.

Judicial punishments are more intense, necessitating the use of a whipping post or punishment horse. Again a fixed number of strokes should be decided on and then delivered.

Less Common Implements

There are a number of implements which are less common in kinky practice, but that can add authenticity and excitement to your discipline scenes. It will be much harder to find people experienced in the use of some of these implements, due to their rarity, but it is possible. Many of these items will have to be made by the user, which is detailed in each description.

Bastinado

Bastinado, also known as falaka in the middle east and jiao xing in China, refers to foot caning. It is a traditional technique of torture since it is very painful but unlikely to leave marks - if it does, those marks are concealed on the bottom of the feet.

I've written it up as a separate entry because while it uses canes and other implements, it is a beast of its own.

Size and Materials

Canes are discussed in detail in the section on canes. Bastinado should use thin canes - junior or senior canes, generally. The thinner canes will ensure that the impact remains on the surface and helps to minimize the risk of damaging the delicate bones in the feet.

Rattan canes are ideal for bastinado, however, other cane materials are acceptable as well. Avoid rigid materials or those that can easily break, such as bamboo.

If you are less concerned about traditional bastinado and simply want to engage in bastinado inspired foot torture, then the use of crops, small floggers, or even thin metal rods is possible. Your imagination is the limit, but make sure that you are playing in a way that won't cause damage to the feet - there are a lot of small bones that could be damaged by deep/heavy impact.

Sensation

Foot caning can be quite painful. While parts of the foot are toughened up from walking, such as the sole and ball of the foot, others are protected and quite sensitive, like the arch. Bottoms are likely to experience the double wave of sensation that is common with canes, just amplified because of the sensitivity.

The arch of the foot should be avoided in general. It is, however, possible to use a very thin, stingy cane in that area, if you are careful. It will be much more sensitive than the rest of the foot and is more prone to damage.

Marks

Bastinado generally will not leave any marks, which is why it was used as a torture technique. If you strike the arch of the foot with a great deal of intensity, you could split the skin. This should be avoided because it will make it difficult for the bottom to walk and is an infection risk.

Technique

It is often a good idea to immobilize the feet, for the safety of the bottom. Bastinado can be quite painful and it's only natural for the bottom to try to move away during a swing. This can cause you to hit a part of the foot you don't intend to, hit at an inappropriate angle or even to miss the foot entirely. You can use various bondage techniques or hold the foot that you're caning if you prefer.

Bastinado should make use of thinner canes, as thicker ones can damage the feet. Shorter canes are also ideal, so that they are more easily controlled. If you don't have a short cane, you can always choke up on a longer one - holding it in the middle of the cane.

Bastinado employs the same techniques as regular caning. Remember that your cane, the extension of your arm, should be making a 90-degree angle with the bottom when it lands. You may need to move around, get higher or lower, and reposition the bottom in order to be sure that your strikes are landing properly. Work with your elbow bent, instead of your arm fully extended, since you will be closer and do more delicate strikes.

Initially, you should strike the heel or the ball of the foot. Both tend to have thicker skin or calluses, which will help to protect the feet. Since most people aren't used to having their feet hit, they are likely to find it quite painful. Get an idea of their tolerance to this activity by striking the ball and heel before moving on to more painful areas.

If you think your bottom can handle it, you can try caning the arch of the foot. It is much more sensitive and prone to injury than the ball or heel, so do so with caution. It can be quite effective to focus most of the caning on the ball and heel, with occasional strikes to the arch to keep the bottom 'on their toes'.

The same basic technique can be used to cane the hands. In this case, begin with the heel of the hand and move with caution to more sensitive parts. The fingers can be lightly caned, but need to be supported (usually with your hand). Avoiding joints in the fingers is important, but difficult to do. Do not cane the top of the hand, for the same reasons as the top of the feet.

Practice

Practice bastinado in the same way that you would practice any cane technique. Select a pillow and secure it in an appropriate place. Make sure that the height is similar to where your bottom's feet would be during a scene. You can draw a chalk foot (or just a circle if you're not artistic), that you can aim at.

Make sure your blows are consistently landing where you intend them to and that the tip of the cane is not landing outside of the circle before moving on to a person. Always start light and increase intensity - a mistake with a light blow is better and less damaging than one with a heavy blow.

Where to Use

Feet should only be caned on the soles, not the top of the foot. Caning the top of the foot can damage or break the small bones of the foot, causing unintended injury. You should also resist the temptation to cane the toes, as they are also delicate and could be hurt by caning.

Positioning

Any position which exposes and immobilizes the feet is appropriate.

Hog ties are an excellent choice because it raises the feet up to a height that's easy to strike. It's also ideal to be bringing the cane downwards, instead of a horizontal strike, since you will have greater control over the cane this way and it's easier to aim.

Ankle stocks or spreader bars are also an interesting way to position the bottom. This helps immobilize the feet and can increase the feeling of helplessness.

Care of canes

The general care of canes is discussed in detail in the cane section. Ideally, feet should be clean before beginning bastinado to avoid getting dirt or sweat on your canes.

Discipline Scenarios

Any torture or interrogation scene is ideal for bastinado since this is where the practice comes from.

Birches

The birch is not generally seen in BDSM practice, but it can be an authentic addition to many different discipline scenes. Used historically in school discipline, it has also made an appearance in judicial circumstances in countries like Trinidad and Tobago. A number of former British colonies have retained the practice that began in England.

If you wish to use a birch for BDSM practice, understand that it will be a DIY project as there are not any commercially available.

Size and Materials

A birch is composed of a number of leafless twigs, preferably from the birch tree (although any locally sourced sticks/twigs will suffice). Twigs should be fairly green, so as not to break on contact. Each stick should be between 30 cm and 45 cm long and only a few millimetres in width. While very small twigs should be removed, larger ones are fine to leave on. Leaves and buds should also be removed.

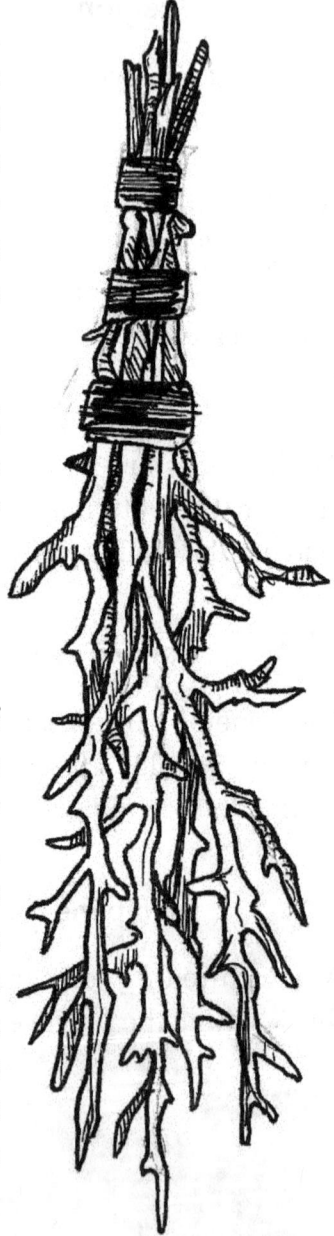

The bundle of 10 or more sticks/twigs is bound together at one end to form a handle. The lashing can be done with a number of materials, from ribbon to rope to leather thongs.

Traditionally, the birch would be soaked in brine before use. This had two main reasons; the first is that the brine would add weight to the birch, resulting in more pain for the person being punished. This also had the (perhaps intended) effect of causing significantly more damage as well. The second reason for the brine was that it acted as a very mild disinfectant in a time when such things were poorly understood.

Soaking your birch in brine is not recommended, it can cause a good deal of damage to the skin of the bottom, leaving cuts which can easily become infected. Sticks and twigs can be dirty and can carry all sorts of bacteria. Brine is not an effective enough disinfectant solution for this situation.

Sensation

Strikes with a birch will be quite stingy and surface oriented, due to the thinness of the sticks used. Since each stick is fairly light weight, there isn't much of a thuddy sensation, even with many sticks.

Birches are fairly intense, although this can be regulated somewhat by the power put into each swing.

Marks

A birch can leave a variety of marks. From rosy, red skin to cuts and welts, it will depend on how harsh the birching is. Expect to see small scratches and red skin at the least. More typically, you will see some raised welts along with the scratches. In more extreme cases, cuts are very possible, which could turn into scars. Typical marks will last a few days to a week, although cuts and resulting scars can take much longer to heal.

Technique

The bottom should be bent over with buttocks exposed so that the Top can get a clear swing. A birch can be a bit unwieldy, so make sure you have lots of room.

There isn't much technique to birching, simply swing the birch so that the bulk of the sticks come in contact with the bottom. Try to concentrate the contact area to the last 10 - 15 cm of the birch, being aware that green, flexible sticks can wrap at high speeds.

Birches tend to be single use implements because they dry out quickly. It may add to the fear and anticipation of the punishment if the bottom is sent to gather the materials for the birch. Strokes can be added for failure to gather appropriate or insufficient sticks/twigs for the birch.

Practice

While it's difficult to practice with a birch, since each one is unique when it's made, you should take a few practice swings before using it. Get used to the weight and length of the birch, so that you can aim properly when using it. Start off lightly, until you feel confident in using harder swings.

Where to Use

Birching should be restricted to the buttocks, but can also be done with less intensity on the upper back. Any area that you plan on using a birch on should be well muscled and some extra padding from fat is ideal.

Using a birch over areas where the bone is close to the surface increases the chances of breaking the skin.

Positioning

Traditionally, a person being birched would be bent over a desk or similar object. Birching horses, similar in many ways to spanking horses, were also used. A spanking horse would be ideal for securing a bottom through bondage.

Care

There is very little to be done to care for a birch, as a new one should be made for each use (unless you're doing multiple scenes within hours/days of each other). A birch should be discarded as the sticks/twigs start to dry out, to prevent breakage.

Discipline scenarios

Birches are most traditionally used in a school setting.

A birching scene could also incorporate elements of judicial punishment or a more general corporal punishment.

Cat O' Nine Tails

The Cat O' Nine Tails, or cat for short, is the most well-known style of flogger to the general, vanilla public. It, rightly, inspires a sense of dread in both new and experienced bottoms. Cats can be wonderfully vicious implements when wielded skillfully.

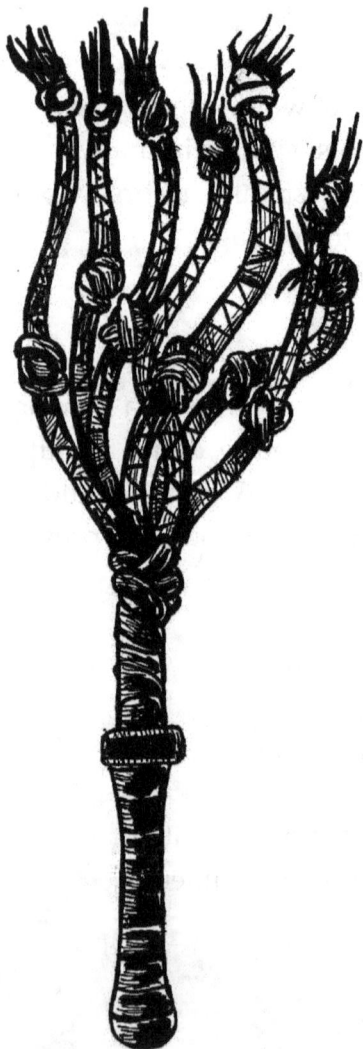

Size and Materials

More detailed information can be found in the entry for "Floggers"

Cats are similar to floggers but have fewer falls. Many have 'nine tails' although cats with as few as two tails are possible.

Traditionally, cats are made with cotton cording. Each tail or fall is knotted, often multiple times along its length. The falls may be plaited or not. The "Captain's Daughter" a cat used in British naval discipline weighed 370 grams (13 ounces) in total, including the handle and tails. For boys who needed to be punished, the "boy's pussy" or simply "pussy" was a smaller implement with five smooth tails, no knots.

Modern cats found in BDSM toy bags can vary a great deal. Some prefer the traditional style, while others have beautiful pieces of plaited leather or colourful rope. Some modern cats have knotted tails and others are weighted to provide a bit of thud to the expected sting.

Some traditional cats are described as being quite long. Modern cats should stay within the same size range as floggers, no longer than your arm. In this case, shorter is probably better, since it's easier to control.

Sensation

Cats are intended to sting and to be intense. Everything about their construction adds to this. Thin falls of stiff or plaited material add to the sting. Knots in the tails add to the sting. The small number of tails adds to the sting. These are implements that many bottoms will hate (or love to hate, depending on preference).

Marks

Not all use of a cat will leave marks, but it is reasonable to expect at least some marking with moderate to intense use. All cats will warm and redden the skin, but that shouldn't last more than a few hours at most. With heavier use, welts can be raised, skin broken or bruised. Some of this is going to depend on how traditional the implement is, how warmed up the bottom is, how tough the bottom's skin is (what part of the body, etc) and how intensely the implement is used. Weighted tails are more likely to leave bruises, stiff, knotted tails can leave welts or broken skin.

Technique

Like a flogger, only the last few inches of the falls should be coming into contact with your bottom. Wrapping with a flogger is an uncomfortable mistake, with a cat, you can open the skin (depending on how close to a traditional one it is).

Any of the flogger techniques described in that section will work with a cat. The results of those techniques may be a bit different, though. Circles and figure 8's aren't much of a warm up with a cat. Warm up, if you want one, is better done with a different implement. Save the cat for the more intense portion of play.

Overhand and backhand swings are going to be the most useful for a cat. You can see a full description of those techniques in the "floggers" section.

You may find that cats are well suited for a style of play similar to cold caning - where the implement is used as punishment (or reward for heavy masochists) without any warm up and with hard blows right from the start.

Practice

Set up a pillow and practice the same way as with a flogger. Your aim and ability to hit with just the ends of the tails are even more important now. Don't use a cat on a person until you are sure of your skill.

Where to Use

Cats can be quite nasty, so it's best to keep them to areas of the body that can withstand a good deal of punishment.

Upper back is traditional for adults and is generally well muscled enough to handle a cat. Make sure you avoid the spine since the underlying bone can make it easier to break skin.

The buttocks were the traditional spot to apply a cat for boys in the Navy and can also take a lot of punishment. The skin is tougher and there is both muscle and fat to provide a bit of a cushion.

If you are confident in your aim, the cat can be used on the chest/breasts. Ease up a bit on the intensity, since this skin isn't as tough as other areas. Be careful of catching a nipple with a knot, it can be quite intense and not everyone will enjoy it.

In all areas, you want to be very careful about wrapping. A cat tail to the face could be dangerous. Wrapping the tails anywhere is going to be quite painful.

Positions

Standing, bound to a whipping post or frame is the traditional way to go. Boys would be bent over with their buttocks exposed. Both work quite well for cats, but any of the positions suggested in the 'floggers' section would be acceptable.

Care

This will depend on the material it's made of.

Cotton rope can be washed with soap and water if soiled through regular use. It should be hung to dry once cleaned. The rope can be sprayed with hospital grade disinfectants for extra sanitation. If you break skin with a cat, it should be dedicated to that bottom, as it is impossible to clean blood out of the porous rope (this is the same for any porous material).

Leather cats can be cleaned with saddle soap or other leather cleaners by following the directions on the packaging. Strong disinfectants can damage the leather, but you can use them if you wish. If skin is broken, the cat should be dedicated to that bottom only.

Cats should be hung when not in use, to keep the falls straight and uniform. If that is not possible, you can roll them up in a towel, much the same as a flogger.

Scenarios

Cats are an implement of punishment, so they're perfect for judicial, Naval or Military style punishment scenes.

When boys were punished in the Royal Navy, they were sent to 'kiss the gunner's daughter' or bend over one of the cannons on deck, with their pants down. The embarrassment of being treated like a small child added to the sting of the cat. While most of us don't have a gun barrel to bend over, the spirit of the punishment can be incorporated into play.

For serious offences, sailors would be flogged around the fleet. The total number of lashes was divided between the number of ships in port. The prisoner was then rowed out to each ship to receive that number of lashes. This continued until all the lashes were administered or a doctor ordered a stop. This could be an interesting scene at a play party if one has enough trustworthy and skilled Tops available.

Discipline

A discipline is a traditional tool used by some Catholic believers for mortification of the flesh. It is an implement designed to be self-administered. It is designed to imitate the scourge that was used on Christ before the crucifixion and looks similar to a martinet.

Size and Materials

A discipline is small and simple. It can be made of leather thongs or cord, bound together to form a handle. The lashes are knotted, so that it's easier to cause pain and draw blood.

Since disciplines are generally made by the user, they can vary greatly in size and construction. A discipline must be long enough to reach the back when flung over the shoulder. A taller person would need a longer discipline than a shorter one. They can range in size from about 8 inches to 16 inches.

Sensations

A discipline creates a stingy sensation, owing to the materials used to make it. Both leather thongs and cord create stingy impacts, the knots add to it. Since it is self-administered, intensity will vary greatly. A nervous or more cautious bottom will strike lightly, a masochistic one will make most sadists look like pussycats.

Marks

While marks largely depend on how hard a discipline is used, certain materials can add to the probability. Rough twine or cord will add to the discipline's bite, making it more likely to break skin and leave abrasions and scars. Heavier materials or weighted lashes could leave bruising. Leather thongs or stiffer rope can leave welts.

Technique

As has been mentioned above, a discipline is self-administered. The penitent should grasp the tool firmly by the handle, with the lashes facing upwards in the hand. It is then brought quickly over the shoulder so that the lashes fall on the upper to mid back. Longer disciplines can reach the lower back, but are harder to control and may hit the tailbone

These strokes are easier to apply to the shoulder opposite the hand holding the discipline. The hand and arm should come across the chest to deliver the most effective blow. It is possible to strike the same side, but many find this to be an awkward motion. Switching hands provides a more natural movement.

Care should be taken to avoid hitting the spine. Skin that doesn't have muscle between it and the bone is more likely to break when struck. Damage to the spine is unlikely with a discipline, but why take the risk.

Practice

It is difficult to practice with a discipline, but one may consider a bit of 'padding' until you get the hang of it.

Wearing a thick sweater or striking lightly will allow you to feel where the blows are landing so that you can adjust your aim as needed.

Care

A rope discipline can be washed with soap and water if needed. Leather should be cleaned with saddle soap or other leather cleaners.

A discipline can be hung, the same way you would hang a flogger. It can also be carefully folded and kept in a box or cloth bag. Hanging is better for leather.

Since it may draw blood, a discipline should be a toy dedicated to one bottom. Since these are almost all self-made, it is inexpensive to make one for each bottom as needed.

Scenarios

The use of a discipline comes with a lot of rituals. You can research some of the specific rituals that the various Catholic cults have used, or create your own inspired by history. Similar tools have been used by a number of different cultures, so there are non-Catholic and even non-religious options available.

A discipline is a great tool for long distance relationships or for times when partners are away from each other but still want to engage in physical play or punishment. The Top can give instructions on the number of strokes and the intensity while the bottom complies. This could be done on the phone, through messaging or via webcam.

Having the bottom create their own discipline can add to the ritual of the implement and help build anticipation. There are a number of ways to create a discipline, suited for beginner crafters to elaborate items that take considerable skill. Even a rope, folded over multiple times with a knot to hold it all together would suffice.

To add to authenticity and discomfort, you can have the bottom wear a cilice or hair shirt. Have the bottom recite a mantra, a statement of dedication or an apology while using the discipline in lieu of a more formal prayer.

Hairbrush

Hairbrushes are intimately tied to parental punishment for many people. They also offer double duty as a BDSM implement, the back of the brush for spanking and the bristles for sensation play. While any hairbrush may do, most imagine one of the beautifully crafted antique brush sets that come with a mirror and comb. These sets can be very ornate, with silver, gold, porcelain or even ivory handles. The bristles tend to be quite soft on these.

Size and Materials

It may be difficult to find an antique hair brush set that you want to use as a spanking implement. Many of these are made from somewhat delicate materials that would stand up to normal use, but probably not fare well being used as a spanking tool.

The size and shape of a hair brush will affect the way it feels, much like a paddle. Brushes come in many shapes, sizes and materials. Today, most brushes will be made of plastic, although wooden brushes aren't too hard to find either.

Many brushes have stiff bristles. Some are beaded with softer plastic on the ends, others can be very scratchy. If you want something softer, try a baby brush, the bristles are much softer and similar to what you would find in an antique brush.

Sensation

Spanking with a brush is much the same as spanking with a paddle. Wider, larger brushes will spread out the impact while long, thin brushes will concentrate it. Don't be afraid to test them out on your hand in the store, but you may want to try to be a bit subtle about it - especially if you're looking at the baby brushes!

The fun part of spanking with a brush is that you get a sensation toy too. When you're done spanking the skin, flip the brush over and run the bristles along the highly sensitized skin.

Marks

Marks will depend greatly on how hard you hit with the brush. Lighter spanking will usually result in red, warm skin that will return to normal within a few hours maximum. Harder spankings can cause bruising. You may even get the odd spot of blood if the bottom's skin is dry and stretched (from being bent over).

Technique

The technique of using a hairbrush for spanking is the same as using a paddle. Please refer to the paddles section for further information.

Practice

Brushes don't generally need much practice. Mastering the intensity of your swats can take a bit of getting used to, so always start out light and work your way up.

Where to Use

The buttocks are the traditional spot to spank with a hairbrush and the best. The buttocks are well muscled and have a bit of fat for padding. You can use a brush in other parts of the body, but avoid using where bones are close to the surface.

Positioning

Spanking with a hairbrush brings back memories of childhood punishments, so the position should reflect that. Over the knee is a fantastic position to give both access to the buttocks and instill the right headspace. Diaper position can add a bit of humiliation to the spanking, which some enjoy.

Care

Care is really quite simple, wash with soap and water after use. Store as you would any brush. Many people find it easier (and hotter) to use their everyday hairbrush for spanking.

Scenarios

Hairbrush spanking lends itself best to domestic situations. Whether it's parental figure and adult 'child', babysitter, governess, etc. there is a strong element of a motherly figure administering the punishment. To heighten this feeling, the spanking could be accompanied by sitting in the corner, waiting for punishment and a thorough scolding before starting.

Martinet

The martinet is similar to a flogger. It has fewer falls and the falls are generally made from stiff leather thongs. It was used to punish young boys in British schools.

Size and Materials

A martinet measures between 30 and 60 cm in total length. Approximately one-third of the length is a wooden handle, simply carved and usually without decoration. The remaining two-thirds are the falls, made with stiff leather thongs. A martinet will have fewer than 20 falls, more traditionally between 5 and 10 falls.

It is best to avoid martinets made with cheap materials, such as vinyl. While it's rare that you will come across any commercial martinet, make sure that if you do find one, it's made with quality materials.

Sensation

The sensation of a martinet is a moderately intense sting. Its shorter length limits its intensity, and the stiff leather of the falls adds to the sting. Since it was an implement used to punish children, traditional martinets can range from mild to moderate intensity, depending on the power used to throw them. Modern martinets can be more intense if they are built larger since they are designed for adult BDSM activities.

Marks

Martinets will cause the skin to redden and may raise some short-lived welts. Marks will be temporary in nature, generally lasting a few hours at most.

Technique

Using a martinet is much like using a flogger. Overhand and backhand strikes are generally used, but any flogger technique can be used with a martinet. Please see the flogger technique section for detailed instructions.

Practice

Practising with a martinet is the same as practising with a flogger. Secure a pillow and practice your swings. The pillow should have a fabric with a nap so that you can see where your blows are landing. Be sure you are proficient with the martinet before you move from pillow to people.

Where to use

Martinets would traditionally be used on the clothed or bare bottom of the person being punished. They can be used on any part of the body that a flogger is used on, sticking to more protected areas such as the buttocks, upper back, chest, and breasts.

Positioning

The bottom would traditionally be bent over a desk or placed on a spanking horse, to expose the buttocks for punishment. While bondage isn't traditional, it can be used to ensure the bottom doesn't squirm too much.

Care

Care for martinets is very similar to the care of floggers. They should be stored hanging or laying flat to ensure that the falls don't get bends or kinks in them. Falls can be cleaned using leather cleaner and water, then hung to dry. For more detailed instructions, please see the care section under floggers.

Discipline Scenarios

School style discipline scenes are most appropriate for using a martinet. It could also be used in religious scenes, as a substitute for a discipline. A martinet could further be used for military or naval discipline scenes instead of a cat o' nine tails since they are similar implements (the martinet would be less intense than a cat).

Slippers and Shoes

While many people wear slippers to keep their feet warm, they are etched into the minds of many as a tool of childhood punishment. Using a slipper to spank saves the hand of the Top and can give extra excitement to foot and shoe fetishists.

While actual shoes can also be used (and would have been in traditional slippering), be aware that the edges of hard soles can cause accidental cuts.

Size and materials

Slippers come in many varieties, with the size depending on the size the feet of the person wearing them.

Slippers generally are made from a soft material on top, wool, fleece and other warm materials are common. They will often have a rubber sole, which is flexible. Shoes can have a variety of soles, including rubber and leather.

The traditional slipper used for slippering is closer to a gym shoe. It has a stiff rubber sole and a canvas or leather upper portion. You can use either type of slipper for play/punishment, depending on how much intensity you desire.

Sensation

Slippers will often make a lot of noise on impact but will have a more mild, stingy sensation. This is because they care made of lightweight materials. A heavier slipper will be more intense and have a thuddier feeling.

Shoes will have a harder sole and will have a more intense sensation. Most will be stingy, but heavier shoes can have a bit of thud to them as well. Be aware that the rigid sides of a shoe sole can be painful in a bad way and cause cuts.

Marks

Slippers will make skin red and warm, not leaving any specific marks. The general redness should not last more than a few hours at most.

Shoes are more likely to leave marks - in fact, there are some boot tread paddles which are designed to leave tread marks in the skin temporarily. Shoes may leave marks in the shape of the sole, marks that reflect the tread or more likely leave the skin red and blotchy. Shoes may also cause bruising with hard strikes.

Technique

The use of a shoe or slipper is much the same as using a paddle. Grip the slipper or shoe in a way that is comfortable. Pull your arm back and strike with the flat part of the sole. Avoid striking with any rigid edges of the sole or the top of a shoe which may contain buckles, eyelets or other metal pieces.

Practice

There isn't much to using a shoe or slipper for spanking. Take a few light swings, to make sure that you can aim properly before getting more intense.

Where to use

Traditionally, slippers (and shoes) are used as a spanking implement, so would be used on the buttocks.

If you want to get a bit more creative slippers can be used on many parts of the body because they are a bit softer. Slippers could be used to strike hands, upper back, chest or breasts.

Remember to regulate the power behind your swing for more delicate parts of the body.

Positioning

Traditional spanking positions would be ideal for spanking with slippers or shoes. Over the knee and diaper position will evoke an image of childhood punishment. Verbal/mental bondage would be more appropriate than ropes or restraints for these kinds of scenarios. Of course, having the Top physically holding the bottom in position would work as well.

Care

These implements require no care other than what you would normally do for them. You may want to ensure that the soles are clean prior to use, or have a pair of slippers/shoes set aside for this purpose only. Shoes may want to be kept indoors and not worn outside. Of course, some bottoms will enjoy the extra taboo of using dirty shoes or slippers.

Discipline Scenarios

Slippers and shoes can be used in domestic discipline scenes. Whether it's a Mommy or Daddy Dominant punishing a little or spouse punishing spouse, punishment with slippers and shoes have a 1950s feel.

Switch

A switch, in this case, refers to the traditional punishment implement cut from a young, green tree - not a person who enjoys both topping and bottoming. Part of the impact of a switch is having the bottom cut it themselves. The ritual of preparing one's own implement can add to the gravity of the punishment or anticipation of funishment. In some ways, switches are similar to the birch, in others they more resemble canes.

Size and Materials

Switches can be made from any sort of wood, although some are more traditional than others. Willow is probably one of the most popular materials for switches, followed by birch. Hickory and hazel wood have also been commonly used, but any strong yet flexible locally sourced wood will work.

Switches are generally cut shortly before use so that the wood is green, This contributes to its flexibility.

In the Caribbean, tamarind is used to make switches. Three thin lengths of tamarind are braided together and oiled. These are designed to be re-used, unlike the single length switches above.

Like canes, switches can range in length from about 46 cm (18 inches) to 92 cm (36 inches), although switches over a meter (39.5 inches) aren't unheard of. Shorter switches are easier to handle, while longer ones will be more painful. Again, like canes, the thickness of the switch will affect its feel. A switch of 6-7 mm (1/4 inch) will feel more stingy than one 10-12 mm (1/2 inch) thick.

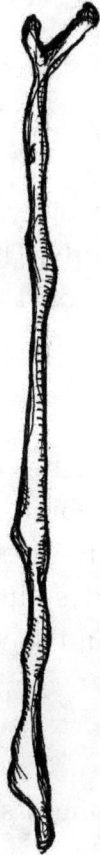

Part of preparing the switch is to smooth out the surface. All twigs and leaves should be removed. The switch should be washed so that it is clean, but no soaking is required.

Sensation

A switch delivers a stingy sensation, much like a cane. This owes to both the overall thinness of the wood and its flexibility. Switches can be quite intense, even when applied lightly. The effects of a harsh switching may be felt for up to a few days after, but generally the sensation fades quickly.

Marks

Switches can leave welts, even with lighter applications. The flexibility and uneven surface of the wood can bite into the skin. These usually resolve within a few hours to days. Cuts and splitting the skin is possible with hard strokes, which could leave scarring in some circumstances.

Technique

Using a switch is very much the same as the harder strokes with a cane. Please refer to the sections on basic cane technique and cold caning. Most use of switches will be in the cold caning style.

Practice

Practice with a switch is essential. One should have mastered the caning techniques and be able to reliably hit their target with a cane before attempting to use a switch. See the section on cane practice for details.

In addition, since each switch is different, it is important to take a few practice swings at a pillow or other soft object to get the feel of it. You may need to adjust your aim depending on the length of the switch. Having your bottom watch this display can add to their anticipation since the switch will make the same 'woosh' type noise that a cane would.

Where to use

A switch should only be used on parts of the body that are protected by heavy muscle and fat. The buttocks and upper back are ideal places to use a switch, although the chest/breasts could also be struck if care is taken not to hit the face.

Positioning

Bent over an object is the traditional position for switching, since switches are most usually used in home discipline scenarios. For using a switch on the upper back, a standing position more common in judicial caning scenarios would work well. Lying positions are also an option, depending on your needs.

Care

Most switches are meant to be discarded after use with a new switch prepared for subsequent scenes. This is especially true if the switch has broken the skin, as there is no way to properly sanitize the wood.

In the case of a braided tamarind switch, it should be hung and cared for in the same way that a cane is cared for. Regular oiling will help to maintain its flexibility over time.

Discipline Scenarios

Household discipline is the traditional scenario for use with a switch. As mentioned earlier in the section, having the bottom cut and prepare the switch can become part of the ritual. If you have appropriate trees nearby, send the bottom out to cut a switch of the appropriate length - whatever length you feel most comfortable using. Using a sharp knife or pruning shears, cut the switch from the tree (this should not harm the tree). With the same knife, leaves, twigs and other imperfections should be removed. If these are left on, more damage can be done to the skin than intended.

For judicial style punishments, the prisoner can prepare their own switch or you can prepare it yourself - in view of the restrained or caged bottom would seem appropriate. Talk through the process or work in stoic silence, as you see fit. As with any judicial punishment, make sure the prisoner understands their 'crimes' and the punishment they will receive.

Quirt

A quirt is a short stock whip, which is rarely seen in BDSM practice. It can be a fun and exotic implement, used for punishment or funishment. Quirts often make a lot of noise, which can be intimidating and exciting for players. Be aware that quirts intended for horses can cause a lot of damage to human skin.

Size and Materials

A quirt is about 60 cm in total length, but this can vary, depending on the design and the quirt.

A quirt has a handle of stiff yet flexible braided leather. As the handle transitions into the body of the quirt, the braid becomes thinner and more flexible. The quirt ends with two long, flat leather falls. These can be oval or long diamond-like in shape. The falls are wider than the falls of a flogger, usually 5 cm or so across.

Quirts that are made for BDSM will have falls that are made of a softer leather. Those made for livestock will be a harder, thicker leather. Be aware that quirts made for livestock are often too heavy for human skin and can cause unintended damage. Even with careful use, bottoms can sustain unintended injuries if the Top is using a quirt intended for livestock.

Sensation

Quirts can range from moderately intense to quite painful. The type of leather used will have some bearing on the intensity of the quirt, thicker, stiffer leather will be more intense than softer leather.

A quirt delivers a mostly thuddy sensation, but stiff leather falls can add some sting to each strike. Often, they will make a loud noise on impact, as the two falls slap against each other, adding to the shock of the blow.

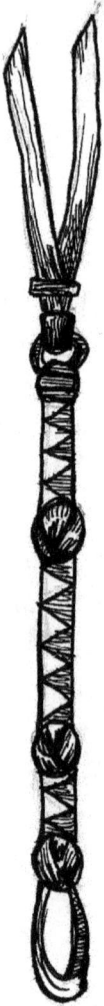

Marks

Quirts often leave temporary marks, reddening the skin the way a flogger will. They can also leave some welts and even bruising at times. Care must be taken to avoid landing the falls on their edges, which can cut into the skin. Most marks left by a quirt will fade quickly, but intense scenes can leave marks that last for days or even a week.

Technique

Using a quirt is similar to using a strap or tawse. While it is a stock whip, it will not crack in the way that other whips will.

The most common ways to use a quirt is doing overhand and backhand strikes, like you, would with a strap or even a flogger. For detailed instructions on those techniques, please see the 'Technique' section for straps and floggers. Keep in mind that the quirt had a flexible handle and is longer than most straps. Adjust your position so that your blows land where you intend them to.

The length of the quirt makes it easy to accidentally wrap around the body. This should be avoided, as the increased speed of the falls when they wrap can also cause damage. In general, a quirt is an advanced implement and should only be considered when the Top if proficient in using both floggers and straps.

Practice

It is essential that a Top practice with a quirt before using it on a person. The aim has to be flawless, otherwise, the Top risks injuring the bottom. The Top should also learn how to ensure that the falls land flat and not on their edges, which is something that simply takes time and patience to learn.

Practice aim on a pillow secured at an appropriate height. Covering the pillow with a fabric that has a nap so that you can see where a blow has landed is ideal. Be sure that you are able to consistently have blows land where you aim before trying to use a quirt on a person.

Where to use

Quirts can cause a lot of damage if the blows are misplaced or used on more delicate parts of the body. It is best to stick to using quirts on the buttocks and upper back (ensuring that the neck is protected). Avoid using a quirt on the chest/breasts, since a minor mistake could cause a blow to land on the face of the bottom, causing injury.

Positioning

When using a quirt, you may want to secure the bottom so that they can not move suddenly. A whipping post would be appropriate. The bottom could also be bent over an object, secured or free, to expose the buttocks. For a brave bottom, they could be ordered to stand with hands behind their head to receive punishment.

Care

Care for quirts is similar to that of floggers and leather straps/tawses. Quirts should be hung so that the falls do not get bends or kinks in them. If hanging is not possible, a quirt can be stored rolled in a towel, similar to flogger storage.

Cleaning should consist of water and leather soap. Good leather soaps will help moisturize the leather as it cleans. You may also want to occasionally moisturize your quirt with an appropriate leather product.

Discipline scenarios

Quirts were not used on people, they are a tool for use on farms and stables - so let that be your inspiration. Any scene that incorporates stables, such as a Lady or Knight scene, could make use of a quirt.

Yardstick or Ruler

Yardsticks and rulers are a simple pervertable. Any store selling office or school supplies will have rulers. Yardsticks can be a bit more difficult to find, but they can be bought at sewing supply stores, some stores selling school supplies and various antique shops.

Size and Materials

Rulers and Yardsticks come in two standard materials; wood and plastic. Both will work for our purposes, so it's really up to you which one suits your needs better. Wood is more traditional but can be difficult to clean and can break. Plastic is easy to clean, is often a bit tougher than wood, but it's less traditional and some would say it doesn't feel as good against the skin.

The length of each will vary slightly depending on which measuring system it represents. A yardstick is a yard, but here in Canada, a 'yardstick' end up being one meter in length. Rulers are often twelve inches in length or 30 cm for a metric ruler.

Sensation

Both yardsticks and rulers will have a more stingy feel to them. They are thin, somewhat flexible implements built of fairly light weight materials. Wooden implements may have a bit of thud to them, depending on the type of wood and how heavy they are.

Marks

Rulers shouldn't leave much in the way of marks other than the expected redness that dissipates quickly. In some cases, with hard use, they may leave bruises or welts. Often they aren't sturdy enough to withstand this sort of use, so may not be the right tool if you want to play hard.

Technique

Rulers and yardsticks can be used in the same way as most paddles. Please see the section on paddles for further information on that style of use. It should be noted that yardsticks should not be held at one end and used in a manner similar to a cane. They will often break somewhere along the length if used this way - especially if you make contact with the bottom in the middle of the yardstick.

Plastic rulers can be used in a nasty manner where they are snapped against the skin. Holding the ruler close to the skin, bend the ruler back and away from the bottom. Let go and listen for the yelp. Be careful not to bend the ruler too far back, since it can break.

Rulers can be used on the hands and feet in a similar manner as canes. When striking the hands, be sure to hit lightly to avoid damage. You should be aiming for the meatier parts of the hands, such as the heel of the hand. You can hit the fingers lightly with a ruler, but again, start light and use caution. See the bastinado section for foot torture and use the ruler in a similar manner to a cane.

Practice

Using a ruler or yardstick is pretty straightforward and doesn't require a lot of practice. You may want to play around with the yardstick for a bit first to be sure your aim is accurate. You can attempt snapping a ruler against any flat surface. I also recommend trying it at least once against your own upper leg, so you know how it feels.

Where to use

You can use these implements on pretty much part of the body. They are fine for use on the same places as paddles and can also be used on the hands and feet with caution. Since these implements tend to be stingy, they are relatively safe to use as long as you aren't going over bone that's close to the surface.

Positioning

Positions will depend on how you are using the ruler or yardstick. For paddling style use, you can use any of the positions discussed in that section.

For use on the hands, standing with the hands outstretched, palms facing up, is a traditional position. For feet, on all fours with the feet pointed up would work well. The section on bastinado will have more ideas for positions.

Care

Rulers and yardsticks can be cleaned with antibacterial wipes since even the wood ones should be sealed. Hospital grade disinfectants can also be used if you wish. For dirt removal, soap and water work well. If you are worried about blood or sexual fluids, it's easy to dedicate the toy to a bottom, since they are inexpensive. You can always but multiple or get a new one if you need to throw one out.

Scenarios

The obvious scenario is a school one. You can incorporate a ruler or yardstick in with other implements for an impact scene or use one for a stand-alone punishment/funishment. Office scenarios can also be a lot of fun, using 'toys' that would be found in the environment.

Punishment & Playing Without Safe Words

Some people require regular discipline and accountability in their lives. Having to meet a standard and being physically punished if you fail is something many of us grew accustomed to as children. There was comfort in knowing if you were good or bad. In knowing that if you were bad, your sins would be forgiven when you had a tender, warm and red bottom. As adults, we don't have this luxury anymore, but some people crave this reassurance from their childhood.

Perhaps common sense, sometimes controversial, when talking about punishments, there are no safe words. Think about it, would it not be simple to get out of an agreed upon punishment by simply saying "red"? If you've agreed to be held accountable for your actions and then want to get out of the consequences of poor behaviour, punishment dynamics may not be what you're looking for.

Punishment Dynamics

Not all BDSM or power exchange relationships will include a punishment dynamic. For some people, this style of dynamic works best for them. Punishment dynamics include a punishment, generally physical, for transgressions and rule breaking. Rules in this style of relationship should be clearly negotiated and expressed. Having a written copy of the rules, on paper or online, is a wise idea. Physical punishment should never replace open and honest communication, rather, it complements it.

If a mistake is made, the partners must talk about it. The person who made the error needs to be aware of it. Apologies should be offered as part of showing remorse for one's actions or hurting others. Accidental hurt is much different than intentional rule breaking and may be dealt with differently. Much will depend on the initial negotiation when setting up the punishment dynamic.

In addition to talking about the broken rule or hurt caused, the partners should also discuss why it happened. Are the rules too strict? Was it an honest mistake? Did the transgressor give into peer pressure? Were they acting out because of some other reason? Knowing why a rule was broken goes a long way to knowing how to fix the situation.

The next part of the conversation should be how to ensure that the rule isn't broken again or that the hurt isn't caused again. Sometimes rules may need to be changed, made more clear, made more lenient or forgotten altogether. The partners should work together to come up with a solution that satisfies everyone involved.

Once that is done, a punishment should be agreed upon. The type and severity of the punishment may be indicated in the rules or punishments may be designed to fit the offence Again, this will depend on what was negotiated when the dynamic was first created.

Punishment should not be an activity that the person being punished enjoys. What sort of punishment is it to spank someone who loves spankings? Either they get a reward for bad behaviour or they begin to associate spankings with negative feelings and lose their love for them. It is usually best to choose something that the person being punished doesn't like, but can handle for the sake of punishment. Just like you don't want to choose something that they enjoy, you also don't want to choose something that is traumatic for them.

The degree of punishment should also be agreed on. You may choose to cane as a punishment, for example. For minor transgressions, a few strokes should take care of things - perhaps under 10 hard strokes with a thick cane. For more serious transgressions, you could increase the number of strokes. You could also designate a thinner cane if the bottom hated stingy implements since thinner means more stingy. Either way, partners should agree to the type, severity, and amount of punishment.

It should also be stated that punishment should not violate the limits of the person. Limits should be respected and not used against someone.

Maintenance Spanking

For some people, having a regular, scheduled spanking or other punishment helps keep them in line. This can be adjusted depending on behaviour since the last punishment if needed.

You may decide on maintenance spankings to happen once per week, on Sunday. The spanking will be delivered with a wooden paddle, 20 swats in total. Perhaps 2 swats will be added per swear word used during the week or 5 swats for waking up late in the morning - all of it must be worked out and agreed upon before anything starts.

On Sunday, the partners would sit down and go over the week. Perhaps they keep a diary of offences, or the bottom is expected, to be honest, and confess their transgressions to the Top. The total punishment is then calculated. If no extra swats have been earned, the bottom gets the minimum. If too many extras have been earned, the punishment may be broken up into smaller parts. A long talk would also be needed to know why the bottom is racking up so many extras.

Some people will use a system like this for accountability, like any other punishment dynamic. Others will use it because they find the idea to be a bit of regular, sexy fun. As long as everyone involved is in agreement, your motivations are your own.

Switching

In some punishment dynamics, all partners are subject to punishment for breaking the rules. This includes the Top/Dominant. While the rules may be different for each partner, the consequences may be similar. Some will switch with their partner(s) to give and receive punishment. Others will have a friend who will deliver the punishment to the Top/Dominant.

While these types of arrangements aren't common, they do work well for some people.

Punishment style Funishment

Some people enjoy playing without the use of safe words and without the ability to stop the scene. It is best to keep this sort of play to people you know well, that you have played with before and whose body language you know how to read. There may be some elements of resistance play involved, where the bottom says 'no' or begs for mercy.

These types of scenes should be negotiated in a similar way to genuine punishments. The type of play, the intensity and the number of strokes (or length of time) should all be negotiated ahead of time. When all parties agree to the terms, and once play has begun, the bottom doesn't have a way to stop things.

This is a play style that takes a lot of trust between partners. The bottom must trust the Top to stick to the agreement and the Top must trust the bottom not to withdraw consent part way through (since they have no way to communicate the withdrawal).

As a professional Dominant, I would get regular requests for this style of play. It added to the feelings of helplessness that the bottoms/submissives wanted to achieve. It also prevented them from 'chickening out' when things got rough (my client's words, not mine). I would always ask why they wanted this style of play. I got many different answers, including wanting punishment for transgressions, but it generally boiled down to a feeling of ownership, helplessness and a loss of control.

Fail safe

If you are engaging in genuine punishments or punishment style funishment, you may want to include a 'fail safe' that will stop the activity. I have often used crying as a fail safe If a bottom begins to cry, I will stop the punishment.

This is just one example and it may not work in all situations. For instance, in a punishment situation, the bottom may be crying before the punishment begins, because they are sorry or feel guilt and remorse for the situation. The punishment will make them feel better, give them a chance to forgive themselves. In this case, saying that crying marks the end of a punishment wouldn't work.

Everyone will need to figure out if they want a fail safe and what it is for them. It certainly isn't needed in all situations, but it does give comfort to some.

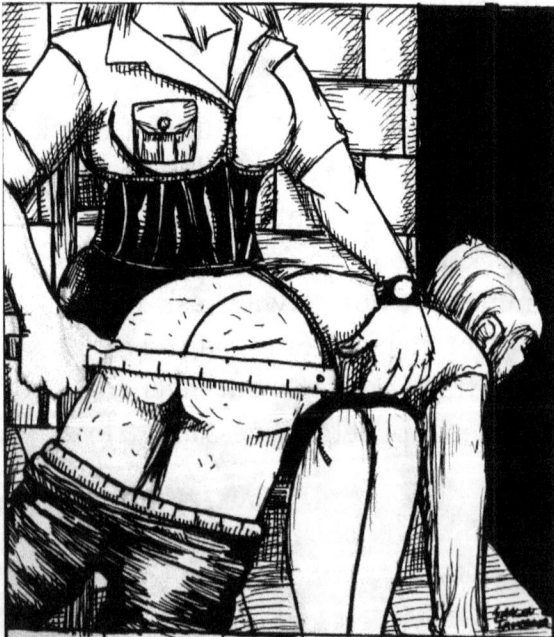

Creating a Scene

Whether your scenes are planned out in advance or more spontaneous, the elements to a good scene remain the same. There are some differences between a scene meant for punishment versus one meant for funishment, and these will be indicated as we go. This is where you can draw inspiration from history to make your activities have a more intense psychological impact, to go along with the physical sensations.

Most of what is discussed in this chapter is for use in play scenes, not for genuine punishment. Of course, there may be some elements that you think would be appropriate for punishments. If that is the case, take what you want from the chapter and apply it in any way you see fit.

Setting the Mood

100% historical authenticity is going to be difficult, if not impossible, for most of us to achieve. We can, however, do many things to inspire the feeling of a particular period of history. Start by doing some research, make some notes about what you think are the most important aspects of punishment at that time. Look at things like historical clothing, expressions, places, and ceremonies.

Use the notes you've taken to figure out ways to recreate the atmosphere you're after. Would your scene be better suited for the unfinished basement of your house (if you have one)?

How about planning the scene at a local dungeon that has the bondage furniture you're looking for? Could you incorporate the idea of spectators into the punishment? Domestic discipline is obviously best done at home, but is there a part of your home that is better suited for doing a scene than others? Do you have a playroom at home that you can decorate to suit your preferred style?

Even if you don't have a space that you can dedicate to re-creating the deck of a British ship or classroom, you can use decorative elements to create the right feeling. If you're doing a scene inspired by history, consider lighting with candles (fully or partially) rather than electric lights. For a school scene, an antique student's desk could become a focal point or a regular office desk could become the 'teacher's' desk.

Thrift and antique stores are a great resource for smaller elements that can help set the mood. You would be amazed at what you can find if you're willing to put in the time. Flea markets can sometimes have great finds if you enjoy searching through the offerings on hand.

If you're the crafty sort, Youtube can be a great source of inspiration and instruction for all sorts of decorative crafts, even some costuming pieces.

Costuming is a fantastic way to set the mood. Small elements can be used to get the right feeling, or elaborate, historical costumes can be created for your favourite scenes.

If you enjoy naval or military discipline, a full costume is fantastic but not needed. You can wear a stark white shirt and slacks (or a pencil skirt). More modern military and naval uniform pieces can be purchased at army surplus outlets. A historical captain's hat can help create the mood you're after.

You can always have a bit of fun with things too. Pirates are popular historical figures, and often employed strict discipline on board their ships. Some of these punishments are very similar to the ones formally used by the British Navy, including the use of flogging. Make use of last year's Halloween costume and show your partner what a 'sexy pirate' can do!

Halloween stores are a great source for inexpensive costuming for any type of scene, especially if you wait until November 1. Nun's habits and priest robes, 1950's poodle skirts, prisoner jumpsuits and much more can be bought for future fun.

Thrift stores can be a wonderful resource for some costume elements. Teacher outfits, office wear, and other costuming can be found at lower prices. You may even be able to find some authentic 1950's pieces.

If you're handy with a sewing machine, costuming becomes relatively easy. There are a number of historical patterns that you can buy, ranging in difficulty from simple to more difficult. There is also a wide selection of Halloween costume patterns that you should be able to order at any time of year. Of course, you can always get creative and make your own patterns.

You can get creative with items already in your wardrobe. For a religious scene, black slacks and a black collared shirt can become a simple priest's outfit with the addition of some white cardboard for a clerical collar. A modest dress in black or white paired with a head scarf in the same colour can make a simple nun's habit. Add a rosary and your costume is complete.

School costumes are fairly easy to create, even more, historical ones. A headmistress may wear a simple ankle length circle skirt with a white blouse. Add lace cuffs and collar to complete the look. The headmaster could wear a tweed suit with a vest, shirt, and tie (bow tie, if you want). School girls, of course, can wear the traditional kilt and blouse, while school boys can wear slacks or shorts with a white shirt and tie. Add a sweater or sweater vest if you like.

As you can see, a bit of creativity can take you a long way. While adding these elements is totally optional, it can add to the fun for some. If on the other hand, you are using these methods for genuine punishment, you may want to skip costuming and creating a fun atmosphere for obvious reasons.

The mood is important for punishment as well, just not in the same way. You may want to have an implement that is specifically reserved for punishments. This way you can pull it out only when needed and your partner knows what's coming. It can help set a more sombre mood.

Preparing for Your Scene

Whether is funishment or punishment, the person on the receiving end needs to know why it's happening.

In a genuine punishment talking about the infraction is important. Discuss what happened and why. Ask for and give suggestions on how to change the undesirable behaviour Nothing will improve without clear communication about the problem and potential solutions. Use the physical punishment as closure or catharsis. Explain the punishment, including when you will stop - whether it's 25 strokes or when the bottom cries. Once it's done, it's done and the bottom has atoned for their error.

When playing with funishment, the focus is less on a serious discussion and more on creating tension and perhaps even a bit of fear. Explain the 'crime', which shouldn't be something you're actually upset about (while punishment and funishment may be similar in many respects, you don't want to reward bad behaviour or encourage acting out). The bottom may even be 'falsely accused'. They may even be given a chance to beg for mercy (if you enjoy begging).

You may want to take a formal approach to announcing the crime and subsequent punishment, or you may just want to toy around with your bottom. This is supposed to be fun, even if everyone is role playing a serious role. It follows the same basic outline as above, but has more room for playful banter, begging for mercy and feigned cruelty. Announce the punishment, again, formally or playfully, whichever suits the mood of your scene.

For a judicial style funishment, you may wish to have a more formal approach, reading the 'crimes' from court papers. A school scene may be less formal but quite strict, with the headmaster or headmistress informing the student of their punishment. A cruel babysitter may, in turn, tease the bottom, taking joy in their suffering.

Once the crime and punishments have been announced, the bottom should be prepared for their funishment. This could involve stripping them naked or partially naked. They may need to be bound to a whipping post or other furniture. They may need to sit in a corner thinking about what's to come while you carefully, slowly, lay out your implements.

The Structure of a Scene

When you're ready to begin, tell your bottom that it's time so that they can be ready. For punishments, you will want things to be quick and drive the point home. Deliver the punishment without warm up and without undue hesitation. This should not be a fun or pleasurable experience for either of you. Skip to the punishment section, since you won't be worrying about building excitement and endorphins, which is covered next.

Warm up

If you begin by striking your bottom hard, chances are they won't be able to tolerate much play. They are also less likely to enjoy the scene if things are too intense too quickly. While some masochists enjoy a rough start, they're not in the majority. Most bottoms like to be warmed up a bit before getting into the more intense play.

A good warm up is for both partners. The top gets eased into the action. If doing something like hand spanking, you will find your hands hurt a lot less if you do a good warm up.

Bottoms will often find they can play both longer and harder with a good warm up.

Decide where on the bottom's body you will be playing. You can play in many different areas, but it's a good idea to take them one (or maybe two) at a time - at least in the beginning. So you may choose to spank the buttocks, which may also give you easy access to the upper back, feet, and genitals, depending on position. Focusing on one or two area(s) at a time allows you to properly warm up that area for more intensity later. Remember, each area will need its own warm up.

Start off with lighter impact, whether it's with hands or other implements. Use the type of sensation your bottom prefers, either stingy or thuddy. This will help your bottom ease into the play and get in the right headspace. Keeping the sensations more pleasant in the beginning makes it more fun to play around with unpleasant ones later to balance things out.

Make sure to vary the location of your strikes, so that you're not landing blows in the same spot over and over. Switch cheeks or sides, move up or down a bit, just make sure that you cover all of the 'real estate' of the area you've chosen. So, in the case of buttocks, be sure to cover both cheeks and the upper thighs, being mindful of the tailbone and sides of the hips.

While variation in the spot you're striking is important, keeping a steady pace also matters. A steady pace will allow the bottom to know when the next blow will fall. The predictable rhythm can be helpful to many bottoms to get into subspace. Think of it like drums lulling you into a trance-like state.

Throughout the scene, but especially during the warm up and optional cool down phases of play, connective touch is important. This is the time you take in between strokes to touch your bottom. Rubbing their skin can feel very nice after a stinging blow, it can be sensual or comforting. It can also allow you to check the temperature of the skin and its texture. Placing a hand in between the bottom's shoulder blades or on their lower back and exerting gentle pressure can be very comforting. It feels heavy, or like they're being held in place - a sensation that many enjoy and find erotic.

The warm up period isn't carved in stone, there is no set time that it should last. Since everyone is different, and people's bodies may react differently from one day to the next for any number of reasons, there are signs you want to look for before moving on to more intense play.

The skin should literally start becoming warm. This means there is increased blood flow to the surface of the skin. Often, especially on pale bottoms, you will see the skin become pink or red as this happens. Not a bright red, nor a dark red, but just a nice, warm, pink glow.

You may notice changes in the bottom themselves. Some will become more relaxed as you get them warmed up, with the tension leaving their muscles. They will lean into the bondage or furniture, often smiling, perhaps getting a little flushed in the face. Some will become more energetic, taunting and teasing you, perhaps wiggling their rear end (or wherever you're spanking them) and egging you on. Since each person is different, it's impossible to give every reaction a bottom may have, but I've found that these are the two most common that I've come across.

Getting Down to Business

Once you've determined that your bottom is good and warmed up, you can start to gradually increase the intensity. Again, you don't want to have a huge jump in the harshness of your blows but steadily hit harder and harder. You can change up implements to those that deliver a more intense sensation too. At this point, you may want to stick to the sensation your bottom enjoys, saving the opposite toys for the most intense part of play.

It's wise to check in with your bottom as you play, especially if either of you are new to BDSM play or new to each other. This doesn't have to be any sort of formal "how does that feel" type of check in. Many people will use a traffic light system of green, yellow and red, so asking "what's your colour?" can get you a good idea of where your bottom is at. Green means good to go with yellow being ease up or close to the limit. Red, of course, is a universal stop or safe word used in dungeons all over the world. You can also check in more subtly, by saying "you like that, don't you?" or "Want more? Beg for it". Of course, you need to find what works for you, the previous just being examples.

If a bottom is new to you and you aren't good at reading body language, you can always do a more detailed check in. Ask your bottom to assign a number to the intensity of your blows, from one to ten - do this before you begin. For this portion of the play, you're aiming for a steady six or seven. Simply ask your bottom what number they're at and you will know if you're where you want to be.

The Apex

Intense play is a lot of fun for both the bottom and the Top. The degree of intensity will determine how long it can last, with the most intense play generally being the hardest to both deliver and take. This is the point in play where both partners are enjoying themselves, feeling great with the energy that is (hopefully) flowing between them and are ready for even more.

For this portion of play, you can bring in more new implements. Go for the opposite sensation. If your partner enjoys thuddy toys, use a cane or other stingy toy for a while. The trick here is to not overdo it. You know you've gone too long with a toy if they start to move away slightly, or the noises they're making change. As you get to know a person, you will be able to tell when their "ouch" is a good one or a bad one (even still, checking in is still a good idea). If the tone changes, go back to implements you know they prefer.

If you are introducing a new toy, no matter what sensation it gives, it's best to do a quick ease in with it. Don't just start out at maximum intensity, start lighter and increase it, similar to the warm up, but much quicker.

This is also the part of play where you can deliver some heavy blows. Keep in mind that when I say strong or heavy impact, I'm saying this in regards to the bottom's capacity to take

A Guide to Classic Discipline

pain, not your individual strength. Some bottoms can't take a lot of intensity. With a good warm up they will be able to take more, but it may be far less than you can deliver.

You don't want to go overboard with heavy blows, so stick to a few of them followed by some medium intensity play. Remember to keep the impact moving around the area you've warmed up, not letting two heavy blows land in exactly the same spot. After their break with medium intensity play, deliver a few more intense strikes and repeat the cycle for a bit.

If you find that you've struck too hard, or you just want to be kind, touch during this part of play can be a wonderful contrast. With a hard stroke, you can rub some of the pain and sting out of the skin with a firm hand. A gentle touch will feel wonderful against skin that is highly sensitized. Of course, you can add to the agony by scratching, especially if you have long nails.

If you want, this is when you can have you bottom count out the strokes for you. Feel free to add strokes for minor mistakes, like missing a number, forgetting to thank you or anything else you see fit. I will often get a bit of banter going with bottoms at this point, which can help me know where they're at with the pain. If they're talking back, I know they can take more. If they're all yes ma'am and no ma'am, I know they're close to the limit.

Finally, you can also change the timing of your blows. Some bottoms will really hate this technique, as it interferes with their ability to process and handle pain, so be aware. Once you've established a steady rhythm you can hold back for a second or two, changing the pattern slightly. What I enjoy doing is pausing for a moment, inevitably, the bottom will hold their breath in anticipation. I don't want to strike the bottom when they're holding their breath (since this increases the chances of fainting), so I wait until they release the breath, then I strike. Sometimes it becomes a bit of a battle of the wills, to see who will break first. Strangely, I always win!

Wrapping Up

Some bottoms will be happy ending play at this point. If you want to end play now, I suggest you tell them that you will give x number of hard strokes with the implement of your choice before releasing them from bondage. This helps you both prepare for the end of play.

For some bottoms, even with the warning, this ending to play will feel very jarring and unpleasant. For them, you may want to do a bit of a cool down before ending play. This is basically the opposite of the warm up, with the play intensity lowering gradually. You don't have to take as much time as you did for the warm up, but make sure you don't rush this either. Increase the amount of non-impact touch as you get closer to the end of your scene. This gives a more gentle ending to the scene for both Top and bottom.

Punishment Scenes

Punishment scenes aren't meant to be enjoyable, so there is no need to take your time building up endorphins and tolerance to pain. Once the bottom is ready, you want to deliver the punishment in an evenly paced, straightforward manner.

You can begin at a strong intensity - again this should be tailored to your bottom's ability to handle pain, not your strength. On a scale of one to ten, you should be aiming for a seven if you plan on delivering a larger number of strokes, or an eight if you are only delivering a few. You can go more intense, but I've found it really isn't needed.

Deliver the blows at an even pace. Strike, count to five to allow the bottom to process the blow, then strike again. Watch out for the bottom holding their breath. That mixed with intense sensation can cause a bottom to faint.

It is wise to either count the strikes out loud yourself or have your bottom do it. This gives them something to focus on and reassurance of when it will end. Don't suddenly decide to add more strokes arbitrarily, since this can cause your bottom to lose trust in you. This is the opposite of the funishment style and for good reason. Most Tops/Dominants will not allow the bottom/submissive to safe word out of a punishment. I go into more detail on this in the chapter "Playing Without Safe Words".

Aftercare

For both punishment and funishment, aftercare can be an important step. Not all Tops enjoy giving aftercare and not all bottoms enjoy receiving it, so be sure to include it in your scene/relationship negotiations.

For some, aftercare may consist of a hug and a bottle of water. For others, they may want to talk for a while and have a snack or meal (I get ravenous after play). Yet others will want to cuddle up on the couch or in bed and feel close for a while. Some people like to use play as the precursor to sex.

Whatever works for you, it is important to express that to your partner. Your needs may be different depending on your relationship with your partner - a casual play partner may warrant a snack and a chat, while a romantic partner would mean a romantic evening together.

Aftercare can help prevent drop, for both tops and bottoms. Drop is feeling bad or a 'crash' after play that can manifest as feeling down, over emotional, crying or just not feeling right in your skin. Not everyone experiences drop and those that do may only experience it occasionally. If you do find it happening to you, let your partner know. You may need to spend more time doing aftercare next time.

Aftercare can also help to reconnect partners after punishment. You can reassure each other that all is forgiven and that life will continue on. The misdeed has been punished, so there is no need to dwell on it.

Putting it Into Action

The skills and themes of classic discipline can be applied to many different styles of BDSM scene. Floggers, for instance, are widely used in all kinds of play from intense scenes to gentle, therapeutic ones. In kink, you are only limited by your imagination.

For Tops: make sure you take the time to practice the skills listed in this book. None of us were born with the innate ability to wield a cat o' nine tails, it takes practice to perfect. Remember, if you don't hone your skills, it's another person - a bottom you care about - who will pay the price. Accidents can happen, but it's your responsibility to do everything you can to prevent them.

For bottoms: Learning the basics of good technique can help you identify 'safe' Tops, at least as far as skill goes. If you decide to help new Tops learn, you can also provide valuable feedback to help them grow. As a Top, I am always grateful to the brave bottoms who have helped me develop my skill set I hope that you have found something of value from this book that will be of use in your relationships.

Classic discipline can add variety and spice to any relationship, whether you use it as funishment or punishment. I have long held a love for many of the implements used in classic discipline, like canes. Learning how they were applied historically appealed to my love of history and role playing. I love creating scenes that immerse my partner and I in another world.

As I said in the beginning of the book, take what you want, what appeals to you and what turns you on. Leave the rest. There is no right or wrong way to do BDSM, only what feels right for you!

Have fun and play safe!

About Morgan Thorne

Morgan Thorne has been practising BDSM all her adult life. She got an introduction to kink through the Queer community in the early 1990's and knew she had found 'her people'. Morgan has also spent nearly a decade working as a Professional Dominant, which has allowed her to expand her skills as both a Top and a Dominant. Morgan has been offering workshops, lectures and BDSM training for a number of years as well. She has a successful Youtube channel where she educates about D/s relationships, BDSM basics and various kinky skills.

Morgan identifies as both a Sadist and a Dominant. She enjoys playing with a variety of people of all orientations/genders/identities. BDSM is an integral part of her personal, romantic relationships. Morgan is both asexual and pan-romantic.

Prior to her work as a Professional Dominant, Morgan worked in health care. This has allowed her to gain a more thorough understanding of health and safety concerns in kink. She retired due to an injury that lead to chronic pain and disability. It also lead to her interest in medical play, a way to continue to use the skills she learned in health care and to find comfort in the loss of a much-loved career.

Morgan has been active in various forms of activism, including LGBTQIA rights and sex worker rights. She is a strong advocate for equality and the human rights of all people.

CONNECT WITH MORGAN

Keep up to date on my website: www.MsMorganThorne.com

Subscribe to my Youtube channel
for FREE BDSM instructional videos:
www.Youtube.com/MorganThorneBDSM

Follow me on Instagram:
www.Instagram.com/MsMorganThorne

Follow me on Twitter: **www.Twitter.com/Nymphetamean**

Friend me on Fetlife: MorganThorne

Join me on Facebook: **www.Facebook.com/MsMorganThorne**

COMING IN 2018

MEDICAL ASEPTIC TECHNIQUE
FOR BDSM

I have two big passions in my life; all things medical and all things BDSM. I have been lucky enough to have the opportunity to pursue both over the course of my life and now I enjoy combining the two.

Unfortunately for me, my pursuit of the medical field ended early when I suffered a life changing and disabling injury during the course of my workday.

I decided to enter the world of professional domination.

As I was exploring this new vocation, I quickly learned that 'medical play' was quite popular.
I also found that as I accepted the loss of my career, I began to enjoy medical play myself. Before, it was work. Now it became an outlet for that passion, which I could share with others in a non-traditional way. I embraced medical play and strove to learn as much as I could, applying my formal training to this new avenue of expression.

I discovered that many kinksters either didn't know or didn't care about the technical side of things. They didn't understand why sterility was important (essential) in some circumstances, or how to avoid cross-contamination.

When I started teaching different medical play techniques, people flocked to my classes to learn. There are bottoms out there who will not play with someone unless they have attended my classes and follow appropriate medical aseptic technique.

It's not as if I have been teaching anything revolutionary. This is standard practice for any medical professional.

As I grow as a BDSM educator, I have more and more people asking to learn these techniques. I decided to write this book for those people, so that they can gain what I consider to be essential knowledge for anyone engaging in many forms of medical play, tailored for BDSM practice. This book is written using plain language where possible and gives definitions or thorough explanations of any technical terms that are used. I want to share my passion for this style of kink, as well as do what I can to help keep people safe. It is the perfect combination of my two passions.

I hope that you find this information useful, easy to understand and implement in your scenes. As kinksters, I believe that we should always strive to do things better and in a safer manner, so that our partners and friends take on less risk in playing with us.

www.ingramcontent.com/pod-product-compliance
Lightning Source LLC
Chambersburg PA
CBHW072227270326
41930CB00010B/2023